Restoring the Body

Treating Aches and Injuries

Fitness, Health & Nutrition was created by Rebus, Inc. and published by Time-Life Books.

REBUS, INC.

Publisher: RODNEY FRIEDMAN
Editorial Director: CHARLES L. MEE JR.

Editor: THOMAS DICKEY
Executive Editor: SUSAN BRONSON
Senior Editor: WILLIAM DUNNETT
Associate Editors: MARY CROWLEY, CARL LOWE
Contributing Editor: JACQUELINE DAMIAN
Copy Editor: LINDA EPSTEIN

Art Director: JUDITH HENRY
Designer: DEBORAH RAGASTO
Photographer: STEVEN MAYS
Photo Stylist: NOLA LOPEZ
Photo Assistant: TIMOTHY JEFFS

Test Kitchen Director: GRACE YOUNG
Recipe Editor: BONNIE J. SLOTNICK
Contributing Editor: MARYA DALRYMPLE
Chief of Research: CARNEY W. MIMMS III
Assistant Editor: PENELOPE CLARK

TIME-LIFE BOOKS

EUROPEAN EDITOR: Ellen Phillips
Design Director: Ed Skyner
Director of Editorial Resources: Samantha Hill
Chief Sub-Editor: Ilse Gray
Assistant Design Director: Mary Staples

EUROPEAN EDITION

Designer: Sandra Doble
Sub-Editor: Lindsay McTeague
Chief of Editorial Production: Maureen Kelly
Production Assistant: Samantha Hill
Editorial Department: Theresa John, Debra Lelliott

FITNESS, HEALTH & NUTRITION

Restoring the Body
Treating Aches and Injuries

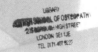

TIME
LIFE
BOOKS

Time-Life Books, Amsterdam

CONSULTANTS FOR THIS BOOK

Josef Geldwert is a Doctor of Podiatric Medicine in the Department of Orthopedics at Mt. Sinai Hospital who specializes in athletic injuries.

Stanley L. James, M.D., is a Clinical Assistant Professor of Surgery in the Division of Orthopedics and Rehabilitation at Oregon Health Sciences University in Portland. He served as medical director to the U.S. Olympic Trials in 1976 and 1980.

Jeffrey Minkoff, M.D., an orthopaedic surgeon, is Associate Professor of Orthopedics and Director of Sports Fellowships at New York University.

Allan J. Ryan, M.D., is the editor-in-chief of *Fitness in Business Magazine* and a former editor-in-chief of *The Physician and Sportsmedicine* and *Postgraduate Medicine*.

Ann Grandjean, Ed.D., is chief nutrition consultant to the U.S. Olympic Committee and an instructor in the Sports Medicine Program, University of Nebraska Medical Center.

John White, Ph. D., is Reader in Human Sciences at the West London Institute of Higher Education, with responsibilities for undergraduate teaching and postgraduate research in exercise physiology.

Myron Winick, M.D., is the Professor of Nutrition at Columbia University College of Physicians and Surgeons, New York.

The following consultants helped design the exercises in this book.

Kenneth A. Allwood is a licensed massage therapist specializing in sports massage. He teaches anatomy, physiology, pathology and medical massage at the Swedish Institute of Massage in New York City.

John Cavanaugh is senior physiotherapist and clinical education co-ordinator at the Sportsmedicine Performance and Research Center, Hospital for Special Surgery, New York City.

Kevin Kennedy is Assistant Director of the Sportsmedicine Performance and Research Center, Hospital for Special Surgery, New York City.

ISBN 0 7054 0716 0

TIME-LIFE is a trademark of Time Warner Inc. U.S.A.

This book is not intended as a substitute for the advice of a doctor. Readers who have or suspect they may have specific medical problems, especially those involving sports-related injuries, should consult a doctor about any suggestions made in this book. Readers beginning a programme of strenuous physical exercise are urged to consult a doctor.

CONTENTS

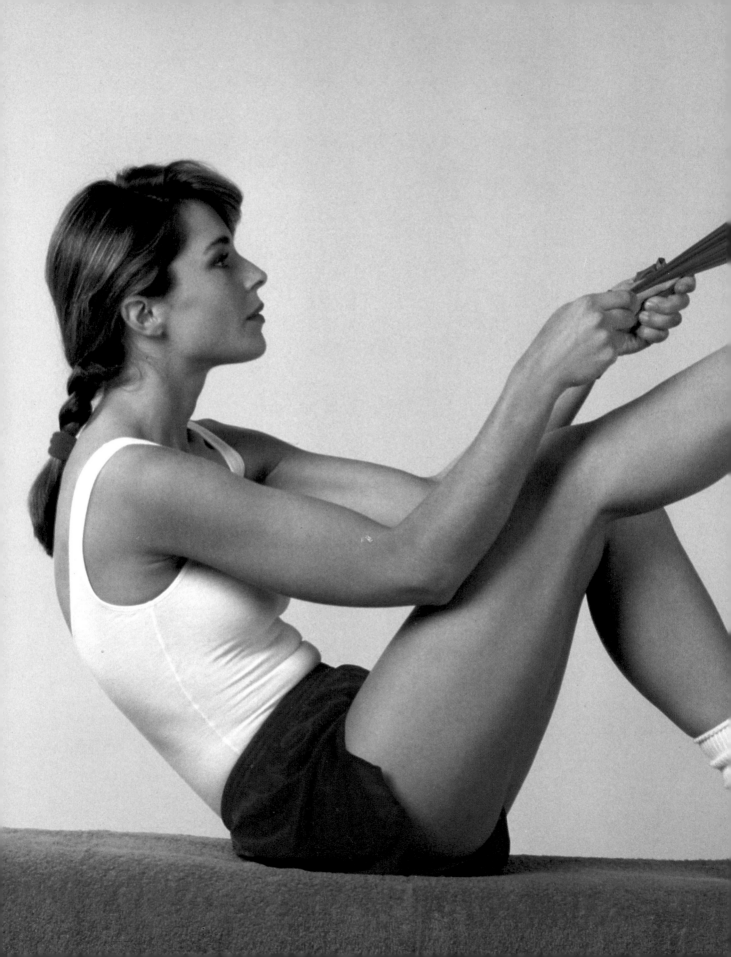

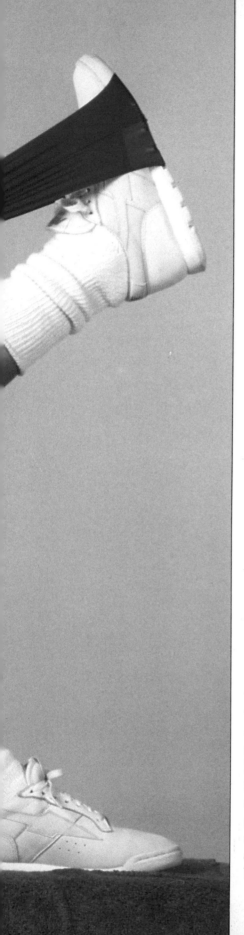

CHAPTER ONE

Understanding Aches and Pains

How and why injuries occur, stress vs. acute injuries, the road to recovery

Public awareness of the health benefits of exercise has produced an upsurge in running, cycling, swimming, skiing, weight training, aerobic dance and other fitness activities. Yet, as it improves fitness, physical activity can trigger a multitude of aches, pains and injuries. Some injuries are immediate and obvious — a sprained ankle, for example. But other injuries are more insidious: they creep up on you over time, perhaps beginning as mild local tenderness and gradually growing worse. Although exercise, if incorrectly done, can lead to injury, the right conditioning techniques can not only prevent many injuries from occuring, but they can also speed your recovery once you have sustained an injury. This chapter explains the physiology and treatment of injuries; the three following chapters show you how to rehabilitate and condition those parts of the body that are vulnerable to injury.

How Injuries Occur: Stress vs. Acute

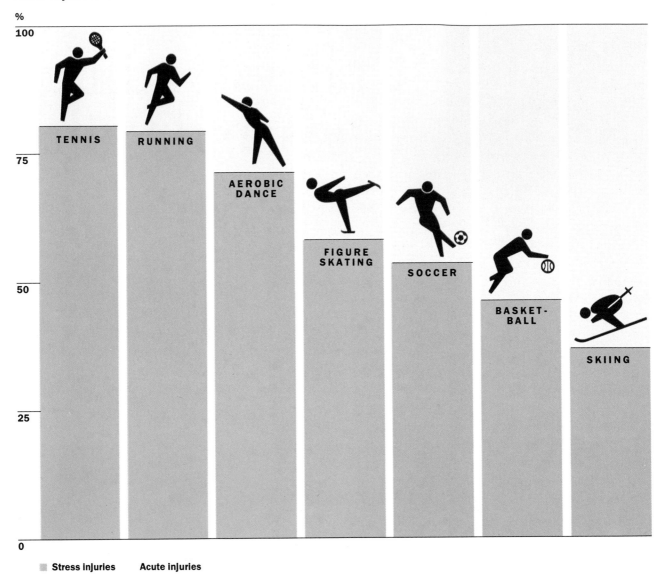

%

100

75

50

25

0

TENNIS
RUNNING
AEROBIC DANCE
FIGURE SKATING
SOCCER
BASKET-BALL
SKIING

Stress injuries   Acute injuries

Recreational athletes and exercisers are far more likely to sustain stress injuries, which are caused by gradually overloading muscles, tendons and ligaments, than acute injuries such as sprains and fractures. In the chart above, based on some 10,000 sports-related medical problems, stress injuries outnumber acute injuries in all activities but basketball and skiing.

Why do injuries occur when you exercise?

When you exercise, you intentionally stress your muscles, producing changes in the muscle fibres. Over time, the stress of regular exercise produces a number of adaptive modifications in the muscle tissue, including an increase in strength and endurance.

During this process, injuries can occur in two ways. Acute injuries are accidents that occur when your body is subjected to a concussive force or collision that produces immediate pain and swelling. Such injuries happen when, in rugby for example, an opposing team's player crashes into your thigh with his knee, producing a bruise, a partial muscle rupture or a "dead-leg". Acute injuries can also occur when a muscle is suddenly overloaded with more force than it can handle. An athlete curling a weight of about 100 kilograms, for example, may rupture the biceps muscle or one of its tendons, the connective tissues that attach muscle to bone. Also in the acute category are sprains or tears of ligaments, the connective tissues that hold bones together. You can sprain a ligament when you inadvertently step into a pothole and twist your ankle. People who engage in contact sports or unconditioned individuals who overestimate their athletic abilities are among those who are most prone to acute injuries.

Regular day-to-day exercisers — those who exercise primarily for aerobic fitness — are more likely to incur stress injuries than acute injuries. Those who exercise regularly for muscle strength and tone, such as weight lifters, are also prone to stress injury, which usually produces pain only after exercise. A single period of high-intensity exercise may damage small areas of tissue, producing a degeneration in the muscle fibre or the connective tissue of tendons and ligaments. These small areas are more sensitive to stress, and subsequent exercise can further damage the tissues over days or weeks: the result is a stress injury. The damage from this wearing-down process may have no obvious cause and generally manifests itself as inflammation of the stressed tissues. When they first occur, stress injuries, also termed overuse injuries, can often be treated with rest and rehabilitative exercises such as the ones presented here. But if they are ignored, stress injuries can grow in magnitude, leading to more serious conditions.

What activities are most likely to cause injuries?
Contact sports such as rugby and wrestling subject participants to falls and collisions, in which parts of the body must take the forces of impact. Bruises, concussions, sprains and broken bones are among the results. The right equipment and conditioning are the best protections.

Stop-and-start sports such as tennis and volleyball, although they are non-contact activities, present their own set of risks, as do such aerobic exercises as running, aerobic dance and bicycling. The potential for injury varies from sport to sport, just as the type of injury does. For instance, while the potential for acute injury is small for swimmers in comparison with rugby players, the risk of a rotator-cuff stress injury in the shoulder is greater. It is estimated that at least two thirds of the injuries in contact sports are acute, whereas two thirds or more of those in endurance activities are stress injuries. A list of common recreational sports and exercises and the possible injuries resulting from them is presented on page 31.

What are the early warning signals of an injury?
During exercise, the body sends a constant stream of information to the brain in the form of aches, twinges and various discomforts. Most of this information can be ignored, as it merely signals that such normal adaptation to exercise is taking place as the accumulation of lactic acid and potassium in the muscle, which stimulates pain receptors.

With regular exercise, the body slowly adapts to these stresses with an increased tolerance for exercise and an improved ability to perform.

The following four symptoms may indicate an injury: any bone or joint pain; severe muscle pain, often accompanied by muscle swelling or spasm; severe joint stiffness with restricted range of motion, such as an inability to flex and extend your wrist; altered sensation, such as numbness or tingling in a hand or foot.

If you experience any of these symptoms, you should stop your exercise activity immediately. If the symptoms are severe or become worse, or if you have any doubts about your condition, consult a general practitioner or sports-medicine specialist. Attempting to "play through" symptoms such as these or masking them with pain-killing drugs may lead to more serious injury.

How can you improve your fitness without incurring injury?

The best way to avoid injury is not to stress your tissues beyond the point where they can adapt to the added workload and readily repair themselves. Begin your exercise programme slowly. Work out on alternate days and increase the intensity and duration of the exercise gradually — the maximum weekly increase should not exceed 10 per cent. Those exercising aerobically should aim for at least 20 minutes of exercise three times a week; a five-minute warm-up should precede each session, and a five-minute cool-down should follow. If you weight train, you should perform no more than one set of 12 different exercises three times a week. A set consists of eight to 12 repetitions, with a momentary pause after the final repetition. Only experience can teach you how far you can push yourself; therefore, during the initial stages of an exercise programme it is important to take the slow-but-steady approach. (Anyone who is under a doctor's care for a medical condition, or anyone over 35 years old who has not exercised for a year or more, should be examined and evaluated by a doctor before embarking on a fitness programme.)

But isn't it true that there is no gain without pain?

Top athletes train at intense levels, often treading a fine line between improvement and injury. They use their pain as a guide to their competitive improvement or as a warning of impending injury. Even those with less demanding workouts can learn to distinguish between the occasional normal discomfort of exertion and pain indicating that an injury has occurred. The information in this book will help you gain that experience. Exercise should not be a masochistic activity, however. Do not continue to exercise if you experience pain.

Fortunately, a large margin of safety is built into the link between pain and injury. One type of pain, called ischaemic pain, occurs when muscle tissue does not have enough blood or oxygen to keep working properly. You may feel ischaemic pain, for example, when you attempt to perform more push-ups or sit-ups than you are used to. In

10 Common Sports Injuries

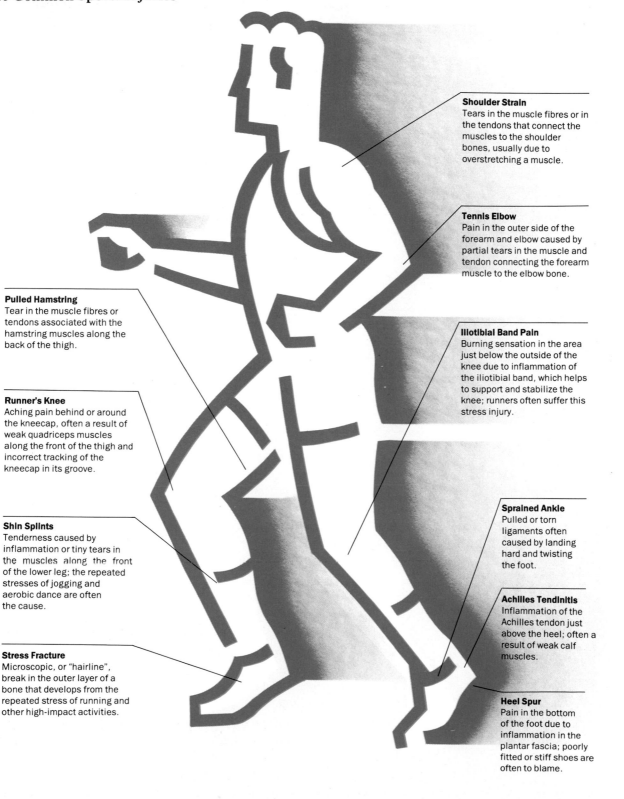

Shoulder Strain
Tears in the muscle fibres or in the tendons that connect the muscles to the shoulder bones, usually due to overstretching a muscle.

Tennis Elbow
Pain in the outer side of the forearm and elbow caused by partial tears in the muscle and tendon connecting the forearm muscle to the elbow bone.

Iliotibial Band Pain
Burning sensation in the area just below the outside of the knee due to inflammation of the iliotibial band, which helps to support and stabilize the knee; runners often suffer this stress injury.

Pulled Hamstring
Tear in the muscle fibres or tendons associated with the hamstring muscles along the back of the thigh.

Runner's Knee
Aching pain behind or around the kneecap, often a result of weak quadriceps muscles along the front of the thigh and incorrect tracking of the kneecap in its groove.

Shin Splints
Tenderness caused by inflammation or tiny tears in the muscles along the front of the lower leg; the repeated stresses of jogging and aerobic dance are often the cause.

Stress Fracture
Microscopic, or "hairline", break in the outer layer of a bone that develops from the repeated stress of running and other high-impact activities.

Sprained Ankle
Pulled or torn ligaments often caused by landing hard and twisting the foot.

Achilles Tendinitis
Inflammation of the Achilles tendon just above the heel; often a result of weak calf muscles.

Heel Spur
Pain in the bottom of the foot due to inflammation in the plantar fascia; poorly fitted or stiff shoes are often to blame.

The Runner's Footstrike

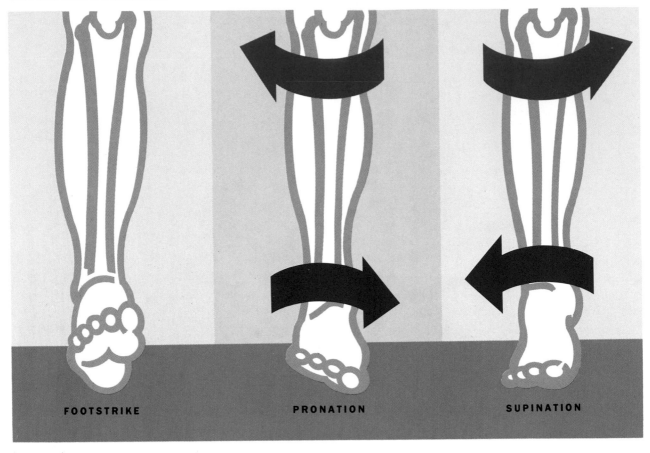

FOOTSTRIKE **PRONATION** **SUPINATION**

The sequence above shows how your foot distributes the stress of running. After your heel strikes the ground *(left)*, your foot flattens and rolls inwards *(centre)* to cushion the shock. This motion, called pronation, makes the knee rotate outwards. As you complete the footstrike *(right)*, these motions reverse themselves: the foot rolls outwards, or supinates, and the knee rotates inwards. Because of incorrect footwear or imbalances in the foot or leg, many people overpronate, placing undue stress on the lower leg *(see illustration, opposite)*.

most cases, the increasing discomfort from performing those extra push-ups prevents you from continuing long enough to injure yourself. In one study, researchers found that subjects who hung from a chinning bar were forced by ischaemic pain to relax their grip long before their muscles lost their capacity to contract. In other words, pain, not weakness, forced them to let go.

Is muscle soreness a sign of injury?
Many people experience muscle soreness during and immediately after performing any strenuous exercise. This soreness is thought to be the result of the accumulation in the muscles of lactic acid and other by-products of metabolism. The pain generally diminishes and disappears once you stop exercising.

You may experience a condition known as delayed muscle soreness one to three days after unusually intense exercise. Common in individuals who engage in sporadic exercise, as well as in trained athletes who compete strenuously, this type of discomfort can last for a week or even more. It is probably the result of torn or overstretched muscle fibres and connective tissues.

Although certain studies have in fact shown that delayed muscle soreness can reduce muscle strength or endurance, there is no evidence to suggest that it results in long-term damage to the muscle or connective tissue. If you experience delayed muscle soreness, you can temporarily alleviate the discomfort by gently stretching. But, according to more recent observations by a number of researchers, a quick and lasting reduction of this type of soreness is actually best achieved by repeating — at a lighter intensity — the exercise that gave rise to the muscle soreness in the first place.

Are muscle cramps and side stitches a type of injury?
Many researchers believe that cramps are caused by intense exercise disrupting the balance of sodium, potassium and chloride in and around the muscle fibres. But no one has been able to pinpoint the precise cause, because the cramps have disappeared before researchers can measure these mineral concentrations.

Cramps are especially common in the calf muscles during or after prolonged exertion. You can relieve cramps with stretching exercises and ice massage *(pages 38-39)*.

Most people who exercise — especially runners — suffer from side stitches from time to time. As unpredictable and as common as cramps, stitches are usually experienced as sharp pains or spasms in the upper right side of the abdomen; however, the symptoms and severity of the pain differ from person to person, and even from one occasion to the next in the same individual.

Although there is no consensus on what causes side stitches, one possible explanation is that vigorous exercise robs the diaphragm of blood, sending it into spasm. Another theory is that gas trapped in the colon, which is part of the large intestine, causes stitches. Whatever the cause and no matter how painful they are, side stitches produce no lasting damage. You can relieve them by stopping your exercise and breathing slowly and deeply, or by stopping, pressing your hand into your side and massaging the painful area.

Chronic abdominal pain that persists after exercise may be the result of something other than cramps or side stitches: such pain should be diagnosed and treated by a doctor.

Why do some people suffer stress injuries, while others who are less fit manage to avoid them?
A healthy human body is capable of absorbing tremendous stresses while running and jumping. Normally, shocks and impacts are spread throughout the entire musculoskeletal system. A system breakdown or injury occurs when part of the body's machinery is not absorbing or distributing stress the way it should, so that stress is concentrated in one area. Often, a stress injury can develop from a slight biomechanical disorder, such as the incorrect tracking of the kneecap in its groove, or a normally imperceptible postural imbalance. Even a subtle

Do You Overpronate?

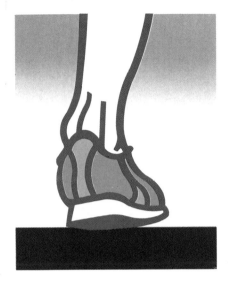

Many runners naturally overpronate — that is, their feet roll too far inwards as they run, putting a strain on the muscles, tendons and bones of the knee and lower leg. Often this is the result of inadequate footwear. If the heel of your running shoe is so worn that it tilts inwards even when you are not wearing it, you may overpronate so far that stress injuries are likely. You can protect yourself with running shoes that are specially designed to compensate for overpronation.

Weighing the Risks

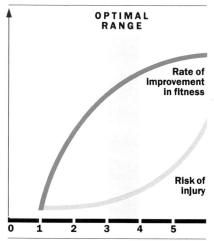

Improvement
in fitness

OPTIMAL
RANGE

Rate of
Improvement
in fitness

Risk of
injury

0   1   2   3   4   5

Days of exercise per week

Although you risk injuring yourself when you exercise, regular workouts have benefits for most people that outweigh the risks, even for heart patients. This chart, based on a study of recovering coronary patients who began exercising, shows a sharp rise in the risk of injury among those who trained for more than five days a week. At the optimal range of three to four days a week, injuries were relatively low and fitness gains high.

abnormality, one that is common among healthy individuals, can result in injuries under the stresses of repeated vigorous exercise. For instance, it is estimated that about 20 per cent of the population cannot properly absorb shock in their feet because of high arches. Similarly, about 20 per cent of the population displays excessive pronation, an inward rolling of the foot on impact that may place undue stress on the foot, ankle and leg. Imbalances such as these do not often, in themselves, cause injury. Usually they must be combined with other factors, such as worn or ill-fitting running shoes or too rapid an increase in an exercise programme. With proper training and equipment, however, many of those with biomechanical problems can exercise safely and, indeed, at high levels of performance. Many Olympic sprinting champions, for example, are flat-footed.

Structural problems that contribute to injury can be difficult even for a doctor to identify, much less the recreational athlete. One of the common complaints that has so far eluded researchers attempting to pinpoint a structural defect is shin splints, pain along the front of the lower leg. Aside from the location of their discomfort, shin splint sufferers have little in common. Studies of such persons show a variety of body types, leg shapes and foot structures.

How severe — or debilitating — can a stress injury be?

In their initial stages, stress injuries are usually not serious. In most cases, all you need to do is rest and reduce the intensity or duration of your present level of exercise until the discomfort goes away. If there is inflammation, however, you should aim to control any swelling (*see pages 24-25*) and start on a conditioning programme to increase your flexibility and strength.

Stress injuries, if ignored, can develop into more serious conditions. At the outset, stress injuries usually result in pain only after exercise. If the inflammation and tissue damage become worse, you feel pain both during and after activity. Continuing your activity can turn a stress injury into an acute injury with increased pain and functional disability. For example, untreated Achilles tendinitis, an inflammation of the Achilles tendon connecting the calf muscles to the heel bone, can lead to progressive degeneration of the tendon, which sometimes necessitates corrective surgery.

How can you guard against stress injuries?

Choose equipment and footwear carefully. A common error that may result in injury is wearing unsuitable or worn-out exercise shoes. Well-designed exercise footwear can help overcome many stress-related problems. Be sure that your shoes are made specifically for the activity you are engaged in: do not assume, for instance, that running shoes will protect your ankles in a basketball game, or that tennis shoes are adequate for forefoot shock absorption in aerobic dance. For tips on buying the right exercise shoes, see page 23.

Besides choosing suitable shoes, you should make sure that you use appropriate equipment. For example, cyclists can minimize the risk of kneecap pain by riding bicycles of the appropriate size with the seat and handlebars adjusted correctly. To avoid ankle injuries, shin splints and kneecap pain, cyclists should wear cycling shoes and use toe clips on their pedals, making sure that the shoes and clips fit. Padded cycling gloves and shorts will help prevent chafing or blisters. Hard-shell helmets should be worn to protect against head injuries as a result of falls or collisions.

Stress injuries may result from training errors. High-intensity workouts day after day without alternate easy days increase your risk, as do dramatic increases in the workload, such as suddenly doubling your running or cycling distance. You should avoid both these practices.

Finally, many activities and sports promote muscle imbalances, which have been shown to be related to injury. Muscle imbalance can occur between two different extremities or between muscle groups within the same extremity. Muscular asymmetry is especially pronounced among fencers: in fencing, strength is developed in the leading leg — particularly in the front of the thigh — for lunging and thrusting, but not in the trailing leg. Promoting strength selectively this way, in one muscle group in one leg, results in a potential for injury in the weaker muscle group or limb when you are engaged in an activity that requires symmetry.

The best way to avoid muscle imbalance is to strengthen and stretch opposing muscle groups and opposite limbs equally. Whenever possible, the exercises in this book are arranged so that those for opposing muscle groups are shown together. For instance, the section containing exercises for strengthening and stretching the hamstrings is immediately followed by a section of strengthening and stretching exercises for the opposing quadriceps.

Can bones sustain stress injuries?

Stress injuries occur not only in such soft tissue as muscles and tendons, but in bones as well. A stress fracture is a hairline break in a bone. This injury occurs most often in weight-bearing bones of the lower leg and foot such as the shinbone (the tibia) and the metatarsal bones of the foot. Stress fractures are common among basketball players, distance runners and ballet dancers.

Symptoms of stress fractures of the tibia are often confused with those of shin splints, although shin splint pain is often diffuse and that of a stress fracture is focused, with tenderness at the site of the fracture. Stress fracture pain usually first occurs during activity and diminishes during rest. Continued activity will make the stress fracture worse, and a localized pain will persist after exercise.

Because stress fractures may not appear on X-rays for up to eight weeks, when the healing process produces calcification over the injury site, they can be misdiagnosed. An undiagnosed and untreated stress

Orthotics — shoe inserts specially fitted for your feet — have been touted as effective in reducing injuries. Studies have shown that orthotics can, indeed, reduce excessive pronation by 10 per cent, which may avert some stress injuries. But such devices cannot prevent recreational runners from encountering such problems as shin splints and Achilles tendinitis that are due to inadequate training, differences in leg lengths and other causes.

fracture — especially of the thighbone or the femur — can, with continued activity, result in a complete fracture. If a stress fracture occurs in the head of the femur, near the hip, part of the bone can be cut off from its blood supply and starve, necessitating a hip replacement. Suspect a stress fracture if pain persists and becomes worse in spite of rest. Consult a doctor for proper diagnosis and treatment.

What is the proper way to treat injury?

For most common types of athletic injuries where pain and swelling are present, you should apply a first-aid procedure known as RICE, which stands for Rest, Ice, Compression and Elevation. For a more complete explanation, see pages 24-25.

If you treat an exercise-related injury with RICE promptly, it is possible to keep pain and inflammation to a minimum. For less severe stress injuries that do not cause obvious swelling and do not restrict your activities, you can probably continue to follow your exercise programme at a reduced level until the pain disappears. Decrease the amount of time you exercise, or cut back on the intensity of your workouts. Perform stretching exercises to loosen tight muscles and apply ice to the tender area after exercise.

Should heat be applied to an injury?

Whether, when and how you should apply heat to an injury is part of an ongoing controversy. Heating the area round an injury dilates the capillaries, thus increasing blood flow and promoting healing by irrigating the tissues with nutrients and removing waste products. Heating will also reduce muscle spasm and pain. However, if the capillaries have not completely sealed themselves following the injury, applying heat will increase bleeding and swelling, causing more discomfort and perhaps delaying recovery. Some experts even assert that you should never use heat in self-treatment unless it is recommended by a doctor or other health-care professional who can give explicit instructions on when and how long to heat the injured area. On no account should heat be applied to an acute injury.

Usually, therapists begin administering heat treatments no sooner than 48 hours following injury. The most common methods are heat lamps, heating pads and hot baths, all of which can increase the blood flow and reduce stiffness. Heat can also be applied to an injury by ultrasound vibrators. Frequently administered in a doctor's surgery or physiotherapist's consulting room, ultrasound heats up the tissues by means of an inaudible high-frequency vibration.

Some people apply liniments and balms before or after a workout. Often made from menthyl salicylate, oils of turpentine, red pepper, mustard and other ingredients, liniments and balms irritate the skin to stimulate the nerves and increase blood flow. Although they produce a feeling of warmth, the heating they create is superficial and probably of little use in the treatment of injuries.

The Hidden Injury: Stress Fracture

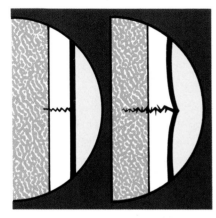

Stress fractures are breaks in the bone that are too small to be detected, even by X-ray. Such fractures begin when the repeated shocks from running or some other high-impact activity cause minute crevices to form in the outer layer of bone *(left)*. Because the pain often disappears after a brief rest, sufferers may return to their sport, adding stress *(right)* that can eventually cause a complete break. Only rest can heal stress fractures.

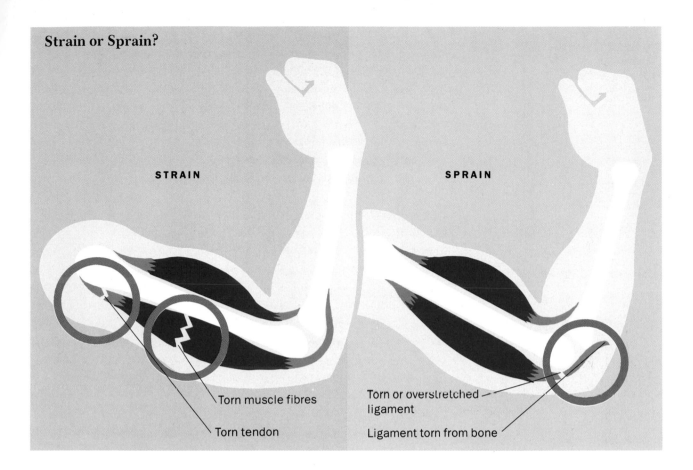

Strain or Sprain?

STRAIN

SPRAIN

Torn muscle fibres

Torn tendon

Torn or overstretched ligament

Ligament torn from bone

Can massage help heal an injury?

Massage can improve circulation, warm the skin, relax muscles and remove metabolic wastes from the tissues. And because it helps break up scar tissue that prevents muscle from flexing freely, massage may also help prevent injury recurrence. Many athletes believe that regular massage helps muscles recover faster from intense daily workouts, thus reducing their risk of stress injuries and raising their training threshold. But only a doctor, physiotherapist, athletics trainer or a certified sports-massage therapist should work with injured tissue. Massage should not be performed on an acute muscle tear within 72 hours of injury or on any area that may be bruised or bleeding. No one with cardiac or circulatory problems or with infections, open wounds or possible broken bones should receive a massage either.

Are whirlpool treatments effective?

Sometimes used in physiotherapy, whirlpool baths allow the whole body to be immersed in warm water as high-pressure jets of air agitate the water to provide an underwater massage. Besides being generally pleasurable, such a treatment will temporarily relax muscles and soothe aches and pains. But whirlpool baths also present hazards. Pregnant women should be particularly careful, since hot, agitated

The names sound alike, but strains and sprains are distinctly different injuries. A sprain occurs when ligaments, the fibrous bands that connect bones to one another, are torn. Usually the damage is the result of an accident such as twisting an ankle. A strain involves damage to a muscle or a tendon, the connective tissue that attaches muscle to bone. Typically, a strain begins as a microscopic tear in a few muscle fibres as a result of repeated stress; if untreated, pain can intensify and the injury can become chronic, resulting in a disability.

water tends to raise core body temperature quickly and can lead to birth defects. Hot whirlpools can also cause temporary infertility in men. To reduce these risks, be sure that the whirlpool water temperature does not exceed 37 degrees Celsius. Besides the dangers of excessive heat, whirlpools and hot tubs can also harbour a bacterium that causes folliculitis, an itchy red rash that usually lasts for about a week. Because high temperatures and agitation promote the growth of bacteria and break down chlorine, make sure that the chlorine levels are constantly monitored and properly maintained.

Don't athletes often "run through" an injury?
It may seem that professional athletes and top amateurs often return to competition soon after suffering from injuries that would keep most people hobbling round for months. Bear in mind, however, that the severity of injuries to well-known athletes is sometimes exaggerated in the media. Also, these athletes are highly motivated to return as quickly as possible, can devote themselves full time to their recovery and are usually monitored by sports-medicine experts who diagnose and treat their injuries quickly. By closely following an injured athlete's rehabilitation, doctors and sports trainers can fine-tune exercises for accelerated improvement. The same injury that causes an athlete merely to interrupt training can prompt another person to stop training altogether. When a recreational athlete suffers an ankle sprain, all too often RICE is applied late or not at all, and swelling continues unabated; the tissues become so swollen that any movement results in excruciating pain. The recreational athlete may seek treatment too late or forego rehabilitation. Complete recovery may take several months, during which time disuse leads to atrophy of the muscles.

Do men and women sustain the same type of injuries?
As a rule they sustain similar injuries, although some studies show that men are more vulnerable to acute injuries and women are subject to more stress injuries. These results, however, may simply be what is known as a statistical bias — men tend to play more contact sports and therefore sustain more acute traumas than women do.

Researchers have isolated some common types of stress injuries for women. The knee appears to be especially vulnerable: women seem to suffer more than men from patellofemoral pain, or discomfort around the kneecap commonly referred to as runner's knee. Women may be prone to more knee injuries than men because they tend to have less muscle mass and looser joints, but not all experts agree with this. Whatever the causes of knee pain, exercises that strengthen the quadriceps muscles along the front of the thigh, the hamstrings along the back and other thigh muscles can help prevent it *(see pages 68-89)*.

Bunions also appear to be more common among women than men. A bunion is a painful swelling on the inside base of the big toe, just behind the joint of the ball of the foot. It forms as a result of the big toe's angling in towards, or even crossing over, the smaller toes, causing an area of chronic irritation at the head of the big toe's metatarsal bone. In severe cases, bunions can produce a disabling loss of function in the big toe, resulting in abnormal walking and running gaits. They can often be managed by wearing shoes with ample toe space and by placing a foam toe spacer between the first and second toes. Surgery is the only way to correct bunions, but is a treatment of last resort.

Women sometimes develop amenorrhoea, or cessation of menstrual periods, as a result of exercise. Athletic amenorrhoea generally occurs among athletes undergoing intense training, and it is often associated with an extremely low percentage of body fat. If you do develop amenorrhoea or an irregular menstrual cycle, whether or not it is a result of exercise, be sure to consult your doctor.

Can psychological stress cause injuries?

No, but several studies suggest that stress can at least predispose an athlete to get hurt. In a study of 97 elite athletes, those who reported a recent divorce, a death in the family, conflict with their coaches or other stressful experiences suffered more illnesses and injuries in a year than their less-stressed counterparts. Among the most common complaints were headaches and foot and leg injuries.

Is it safe to use drugs for quick pain relief?

Aspirin is the drug most frequently recommended for pain relief. It is cheap, available without a prescription and relatively safe, and in addition to its pain-killing properties, it is a mild but effective anti-inflammatory medication: it reduces swelling and so further alleviates pain. However, it may irritate the stomach lining. Also, since aspirin is an anti-coagulant and impairs blood clotting, do not take it if you may have severe repetitive traumas and bleeding.

If you are injured, you should take aspirin in addition to — but not instead of — practising RICE. Aspirin is especially useful for relieving the pain and inflammation of tendinitis. Six aspirins a day — two with every meal — is a common dosage, but do not take it immediately before you exercise, as it may mask pain symptomatic of injury.

Acetaminophen, an aspirin substitute that will not upset your stomach, has pain-killing effects similar to those of aspirin, but it has no anti-inflammatory effect. The usual dosage is two tablets every four to six hours. Ibuprofen, another aspirin substitute, has similar effects to aspirin's in reducing pain and inflammation; it has fewer side effects but is more expensive than aspirin.

Many other pain-killing drugs are available by prescription from a doctor. These drugs should be used only under strict medical supervision. Prescription drugs such as anaesthetics, narcotics or analgesics should never be used in conjunction with intense exercise or competition, since these substances will mask pain and may allow you to injure yourself seriously as a result.

A s participation in sports and exercise programmes increases, so does the number of reported exertional headaches — brief, intense headaches that begin shortly after strenuous physical activity. Fewer than 1 per cent of these headaches have a serious underlying physical cause. To cure an exertional headache, simply reduce your level of activity until the headache goes away. If headaches persist, however, you should consult a doctor.

When should you see a doctor?

If you wonder whether or not you should see a doctor, you probably should. Experience and common sense will usually tell you which aches and pains need medical care; any sudden, severe pain is a sign that something is wrong and needs attention. Pain is not always a reliable indicator of injury, however. For sports injuries, there are some special indications that you should see a doctor. Any injury to a joint or the ligaments around it, especially an injury that restricts its motion, indicates that you should keep the joint immobilized until you can see a doctor. And any injury that fails to heal, whether or not it involves a joint, requires medical attention. Any sign that an infection has developed, such as a fever or the appearance of pus, means that you should seek treatment as soon as possible.

What kind of doctor should you see for treatment of sports injuries?

Prompt, effective treatment of sports injuries is available from a wide variety of sources. These include general practitioners, physiotherapists, osteopaths, chiropodists and a host of trainers, coaches, sports psychologists and nutritionists who work with athletes. As participation in recreational sports and exercise activities has grown, so has the number of practitioners in the field of sports medicine.

There are three main types of sports-injury clinic in the United Kingdom: National Health Service (NHS) clinics, private multi-disciplinary clinics and private physiotherapy clinics. NHS clinics will treat patients free of charge, but may require a doctor's referral letter. It may, however, be advisable to check with the hospital about likely waiting time for an appointment. Both types of private clinic charge for treatment, but most will see patients immediately or within a few days. The Sports Council in London and its regional offices are able to provide information on all types of sports-injury clinics. Athletics clubs and associations may also be able to steer you to experienced sports-medicine specialists.

Since it can be difficult for the recreational athlete to differentiate aches and pains from potentially serious injuries, diagnosis of all but the most trivial injuries is best done by a doctor who has had experience with injured athletes. Frequently, a specialist will prescribe rehabilitative exercises to eliminate the cause of your injury and to get you back into shape for continued activity. If a doctor simply packs your injured joint in ice, however, and tells you to rest for a few days, you may not be getting proper care or attention.

Given the chance of injury, isn't it safer not to exercise?

A commitment to an exercise programme is increasingly seen by doctors as necessary for maintaining both physical and emotional health. Many ailments associated with ageing, for instance, are actually symptoms of a sedentary lifestyle: obesity, reduction of bone mineral content, elevated blood pressure and serum cholesterol levels, slower

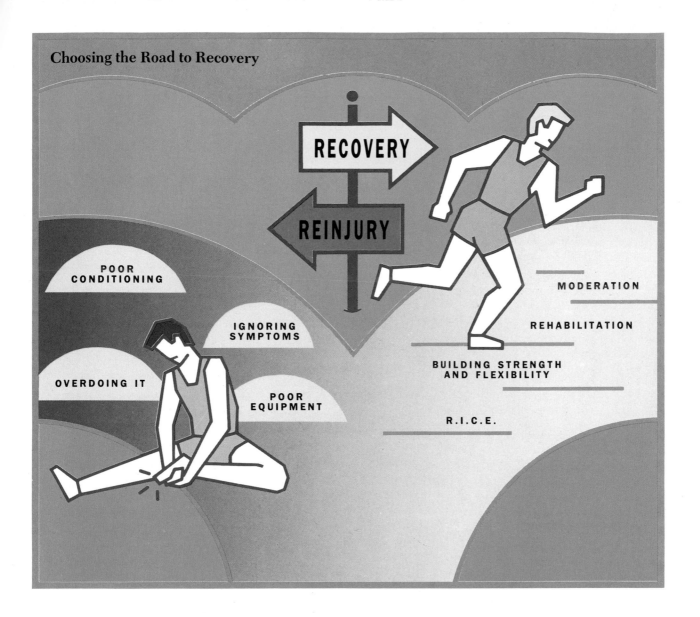

reflexes, smaller range of joint motion, higher stress levels, anxiety, depression, and reduced aerobic capacity. Studies indicate that regular exercise may be associated with a reduced risk of cardiovascular disease, hypertension and stroke. New evidence also shows that those who exercise and maintain an active lifestyle throughout their lives tend to live longer than those who remain sedentary.

Weighed against the benefits of exercise, an occasional case of shin splints or Achilles tendinitis seems trivial. Most injuries do not seem trivial when you have them, however. The remaining pages in this chapter will help you to identify the injuries related to your chosen activities, provide guidelines for treating them and offer ways in which to prevent them from recurring.

Studies show that exercisers who become injured tend to reinjure themselves. Among the reasons are poor conditioning and overdoing an activity before injured tissue has a chance to heal. To ensure proper recovery from stress injuries, you should first apply RICE (Rest, Ice, Compression and Elevation), as explained on pages 24-25. Then exercise moderately and undertake a strength and flexibility programme to prevent reinjury.

How to Design Your Own Programme

An occasional ache or bout of soreness that accompanies exercise is usually not a problem; in fact, it is one indicator that your body is adapting itself to exercise. But a recurring ache or pain or an increase in severity of pain may signal that an injury has occurred. In order to recover from stress injuries, or to prevent them from happening in the first place, you need to assess your approach to exercise and see if you are unwittingly increasing your risk of injury. Start by answering the questions on these two pages.

Are you injury-prone?

1 What shape are you in?

Being in good physical condition not only benefits your health and appearance, it also helps you avoid the kinds of injuries described in this book. Muscular strength and endurance, two of the cornerstones of fitness, help protect you against the sudden strains that can happen in any physical activity, and especially in sports. Flexibility, a third aspect of being fit, protects you against damage from sudden movements outside the usual range of your joints. And aerobic endurance, the body's ability to deliver oxygen to working muscles, helps keep you from experiencing excessive fatigue. So, if you have been inactive, start an exercise programme that will gradually build up your strength, flexibility and aerobic endurance.

2 How old are you?

As most people age, they experience some deterioration in strength, flexibility and endurance; however, regular exercise can offset most of the increased risk of injury that these changes pose. In fact, some researchers believe that 50 per cent or more of the loss of flexibility and endurance that occurs between the ages of 30 and 70 may be the result of inactivity rather than ageing. The best way to avoid injury as you get older, therefore, is not to take it easy, but to exercise regularly. Your programme should include exercises such as the ones presented in this book, which condition those parts of the body most heavily used in the activities you pursue.

3 Are you a weekend athlete?

Bouts of intense exercise at weekends — several demanding sets of tennis, for example — stress your muscles and tendons, but do little to condition them. This increases your chances of injury. Researchers have confirmed that you can build strength and endurance only by exercising at least three times a week. So to avoid being injury-prone at weekends, you should begin an exercise programme that you carry on during the week. Ideally, you should combine an aerobic exercise such as running or swimming with stretching and strengthening exercises that condition the muscles you use in your weekend sport. For a sport-by-sport guide, see page 31.

4 Do you approach an exercise programme with a do-or-die attitude?

Exercise is among the safest, most reliable methods of reducing stress and decreasing the risk of heart disease. Some people, however, manage to turn exercise itself into a form of stress, increasing their chances of illness and injury. Such people approach exercise with the same obsessive, harried attitude they bring to bear on all their daily activities, pressing themselves constantly to run harder, swim faster or lift more weight. Rather than always trying to surpass your own performance and that of everyone round you, expect to improve your fitness gradually and in small increments, especially if you are out of shape to start with. Forcing improvement by pushing yourself to the point of pain will only increase your chances of injury.

5 | Do you warm up properly before you exercise?

Studies have shown that warming up muscles before exercise helps protect them from injury, since cold muscles are less elastic and therefore more susceptible to tearing. Many people stretch to warm up, but stretching does not warm up a muscle. Before any vigorous exercise, you should first perform an aerobic activity such as jogging at a slow pace to get blood flowing to all your muscles and joints. A muscle's elasticity increases as it becomes suffused with blood, thereby reducing the risk of tearing.

You can follow a warm-up with a stretching routine, which is an excellent safeguard against injury if done properly. One major survey of runners found that a significant proportion of their reported injuries was related to the wrong sort of stretching. Ballistic stretches, which use the weight and momentum of a body part to stretch a muscle, such as kicking a leg to stretch the hamstrings, are particularly hazardous. Another common stretching technique that can cause harm is toe-touching with locked knees. The stretches in this book are designed to stretch your muscles slowly and gradually, both to prevent injury and to help your muscles recover if you become injured.

6 | Do you ignore aches and pains?

Despite what you may have heard about professional athletes who continue playing while injured, sports-medicine specialists agree that rest is needed for most injuries to heal. If a muscle or joint hurts, do not use it. What allows top-level athletes to return to play so quickly after an injury is not gritting their teeth and ignoring the pain, but rather swift, expert attention to the injury — beginning with Rest, Ice, Compression and Elevation, or RICE (*pages 24-25*). Exercising before an injury has been properly treated and before the pain and swelling have ceased not only worsens the injury, but can lead to altered body movements, such as limping, which can cause reinjury or produce other stress injuries. The strengthening and stretching conditioners in this book will allow you to return to your favourite sports activities as quickly as possible and without risking reinjury.

Are you wearing the correct shoe?

One of the most important decisions you can make before embarking on an exercise programme or playing a sport is what kind of shoe you will wear. The most expensive shoes, or those with the most cushioning, are not necessarily the best for your activity. Studies show that regardless of the price of the shoe or the materials it is made of, all shoes will lose from 25 to 50 per cent of their resilience long before they appear worn out. Replace shoes when they have lost their bounce or when the heel supports begin to collapse.

Match the shoes you wear with the activity for which they are intended. Running shoes, for example, are designed for forward motion and not for the side-to-side movement and quick stops and starts involved in aerobic dance, tennis or basketball. If you wear running shoes during these activities, you run the risk of injuring your ankles.

Your shoes should be snug in width and long enough to ensure your toes do not touch the front. Make sure, too, that your heel is held firmly in place.

RICE: The First Line of Defence

The best form of immediate treatment for almost any sports-related injury is RICE, which is an acronym for Rest, Ice, Compression and Elevation. As shown in the chart opposite, these measures should be taken when the injury occurs and continued for as long as pain and swelling persist.

Rest means immobilizing the injured body part — keeping weight off a sprained ankle, for example. For less serious stress injuries, or simple muscle aches resulting from overexertion, rest can simply be a temporary halt or reduction in your exercise level. For most injuries, rest generally means taking it easy until the pain goes away.

Most injuries that are sports related respond well to ice, which acts as a local anaesthetic, slows blood flow to the area and reduces swelling. If the injury is near the surface, you can rub ice lightly over the affected part. For deeper injuries involving joint pain, you can wrap a towel round crushed ice and apply it to the injured body part.

The third component of the RICE prescription is compression, which usually involves wrapping an elastic bandage round the injured area. Apply compression whenever there is swelling to help slow the accumulation of fluids in the tissues and allow for a more speedy recovery. The bandage should be snug but not tight. Often, you can apply ice and compression at the same time: put crushed ice in a towel, apply it to the injury site and hold it in place with an elastic bandage.

Finally, when there is swelling, elevate the injured area. If the body part is kept raised, gravity will help keep excess blood and fluids away from the injury site. Elevation is particularly important for ankle sprains and conditions that produce swelling near the end of an extremity.

When treating yourself or someone else with RICE, remove the ice and unwrap the elastic bandage every half hour so that blood circulation is not impaired. Wait for approximately 15 minutes before you reapply both bandage and ice.

The chart opposite shows how long to continue each type of treatment and when you should start exercising again. Simple stretches come first; muscle-building and aerobic routines should wait until you are back to 75 per cent of your previous level of strength. To avoid reinjury, always stop exercising when you feel pain.

From Injury to Recovery

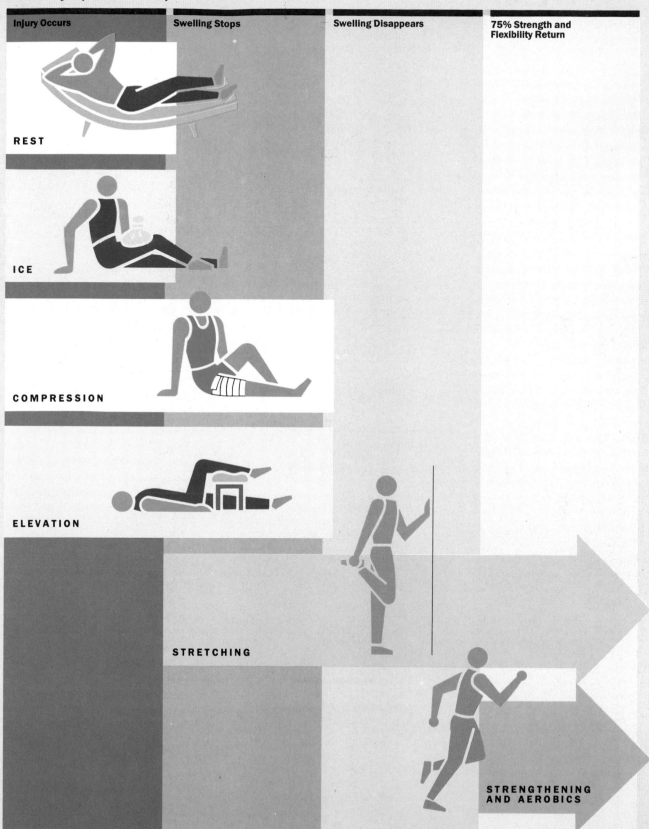

Injury Occurs	Swelling Stops	Swelling Disappears	75% Strength and Flexibility Return

REST

ICE

COMPRESSION

ELEVATION

STRETCHING

STRENGTHENING AND AEROBICS

A Prevention and Recovery Guide

Each injury in this chart is followed by tips for preventing the injury, then by suggestions to speed recovery. The exercises in this book will do both. For most of these injuries, the first step to recovery is to apply RICE: Rest, Ice, Compression and Elevation *(see chart, page 25)*. If you have any questions about the nature or severity of your injury, consult a doctor promptly.

INJURY/SYMPTOMS	PREVENTION AND RECOVERY TIPS
Achilles tendinitis Tightness or pain from lower calf to heel, especially when walking fast or jogging	Do not run strenuously or walk briskly uphill; stretch carefully and strengthen calf muscles *Exercises: pages 52-55*
Black toenail Discoloration caused by blood under toenail	Ask a doctor to puncture nail to relieve pressure and prevent loss of nail; choose exercise shoes with adequate toe room and a firm heel cup to prevent the foot from sliding forwards
Blister Swollen, fluid-filled bubble in skin	Pop and drain blister with sterile needle; choose exercise shoes with adequate toe room and firm heel counter, wear clean socks; do not place tape on vulnerable areas; protect red, swollen areas before blisters develop
Bunion Bony protrusion at base of big toe; foot pain and stiffness; big toe turned inwards	Choose sports shoes with plenty of toe room and arch supports; do not wear tight-fitting socks or high-heeled shoes; consult doctor
Bursitis Pain, tenderness and swelling of affected joint; restriction of its normal motion	Warm up properly; wear warm clothing in cold weather to protect affected joint; protect joint with padding
Cuboid bone displacement Diffuse pain and tenderness at the outside of ankle, especially when walking barefoot	Choose proper running shoes; some recurrent cases may be helped by orthotics (contoured plates put in shoes to control and support feet); if pain persists, see a chiropodist
Heel spur Pain and swelling just under heelbone	Choose proper exercise shoes; fit arch supports in shoes if needed; stretch and strengthen calf muscles *Exercises: pages 52-55*
Iliotibial band pain Pain, sometimes radiating up the outside of thigh; tenderness at outside of knee	Choose proper running shoes to control excessive pronation; do not run downhill or in the same direction on graded roads for long periods *Exercises: pages 90-91*
Jumper's knee Pain at bottom of kneecap; weakness of leg in severe cases	Use knee brace to aid recovery; may need surgical treatment if chronic; strengthen and stretch quadriceps *Exercises: pages 72-77*
Lower back pain Pain when bending or stretching back; muscle spasm and swelling of back muscles	Warm up carefully; do not arch back when lifting or standing up; see doctor if pain persists; strengthen abdominal muscles; exercise to develop flexibility of back, hip and thigh muscles *Exercises: pages 68-71, 78-83, 116-119*
Muscle cramps Painful, involuntary contraction of muscles, often of the calf	Briefly stretch; massage cramping muscles gently to relieve pain; drink fluid before and during exercise; do not take medication that may induce cramps
Muscle soreness Diffuse pain and sometimes swelling of a muscle	Warm up and stretch carefully; do not suddenly increase training intensity or run excessively on hard surfaces or downhill

INJURY/SYMPTOMS	PREVENTION AND RECOVERY TIPS
Pulled hamstrings Pain in back of thigh when moving or stretching leg; swelling and loss of strength in upper leg	Warm up carefully; strengthen hamstring muscles and stretch hamstrings and quadriceps muscles *Exercises: pages 68-77*
Runner's knee Aching pain behind or around kneecap	Choose proper running shoes and, if needed, orthotics; increase strength and flexibility of quadriceps muscles *Exercises: pages 72-77*
Sciatica Tingling or numbness in small toes and outside of feet; pain or cramping in buttocks or outer thighs	Do not run down steep hills; stretch lower back and hip muscles; consult doctor if pain persists *Exercises: pages 118-119*
Shin splints Discomfort or burning pain in shin or calf	Do not run on concrete or uneven terrain; warm up carefully; choose proper sports shoes; consult doctor if pain persists (injury may be a stress fracture) *Exercises: pages 52-57*
Shoulder strain Pain when moving or stretching shoulder; swelling of shoulder and loss of strength	Warm up properly; stretch and strengthen shoulder muscles *Exercises: pages 108-115*
Side stitch Muscle cramp usually in upper right abdomen	Take deep breaths and massage affected area; do not exercise vigorously immediately following a meal; avoid constipation
Skier's thumb Sudden, severe pain in thumb after a fall or collision; feeling of popping or tearing; swelling, tenderness and discoloration may appear	Use strapless ski poles; tape thumb to aid recovery and prevent reinjury; consult doctor
Sprained ankle Pain and swelling of ankle; may be painful to bear weight on foot and ankle	Tape ankle to aid recovery and prevent reinjury; warm up carefully; strengthen muscles of lower leg and foot; consult doctor if your ankle cannot bear weight — may be tendon rupture or bone fracture *Exercises: pages 46-51*
Sprained wrist Sudden, severe pain in wrist after a fall or collision; feeling of popping or tearing, swelling, tenderness and discoloration	Warm up carefully; tape wrist after recovery to prevent reinjury; consult doctor for X-ray examination of wrist, which may be fractured; strengthen muscles of hand and forearm *Exercises: pages 100-103*
Stress fracture Dull ache that persists after exercise; mild swelling and tenderness	Choose proper footwear; do not suddenly increase intensity or duration of exercise; if you suspect a stress fracture, see a doctor — persistent shin splints may indicate a stress fracture (see *shin splints*)
Tennis elbow Pain on outside of elbow, especially when gripping and twisting; weak grip	Improve tennis technique, especially backhand strokes; warm up carefully before playing; do not string racket too tightly; strengthen muscles of forearm and hand *Exercises: pages 100-103*

The Hazards of Heat and Cold

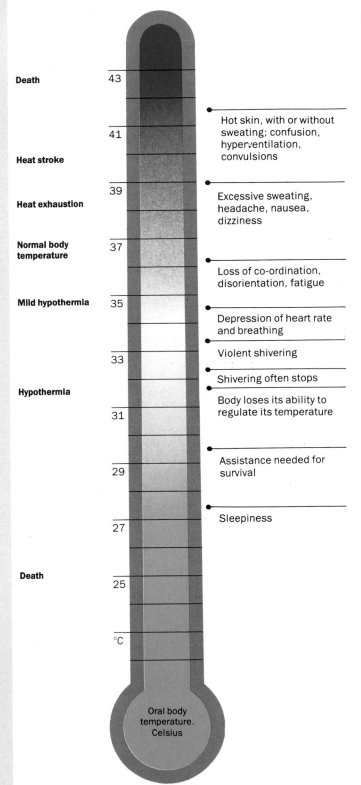

Death — 43

— 41

Heat stroke

— 39

Heat exhaustion

Normal body temperature — 37

Mild hypothermia — 35

— 33

Hypothermia

— 31

— 29

— 27

Death

— 25

°C

Oral body temperature. Celsius

Hot skin, with or without sweating; confusion, hyperventilation, convulsions

Excessive sweating, headache, nausea, dizziness

Loss of co-ordination, disorientation, fatigue

Depression of heart rate and breathing

Violent shivering

Shivering often stops

Body loses its ability to regulate its temperature

Assistance needed for survival

Sleepiness

You are more susceptible to heat injury if you are: obese • unfit • dehydrated • not used to the heat • ill • under 15 or over 40

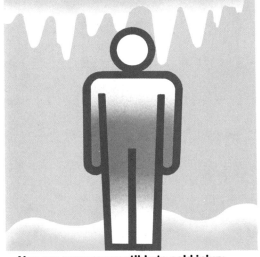

You are more susceptible to cold injury if you: are thin • are ill or injured • are wet • have consumed alcohol or drugs • are under 15 or over 40 • have used ice or snow to relieve thirst

Exercising in Heat and Cold

When your body's internal temperature begins to rise, the "thermostat" in the brain initiates changes in body functions to radiate heat away from your trunk. Without this regulating mechanism, even a 2-kilometre run could cause your working muscles to raise your body temperature by more than 1.5 degrees Celsius.

Sweating is the main way in which heat is dissipated; evaporation cools your skin and the blood that flows to it. For this reason, drinking enough fluids is essential to avoid heat injury. But thirst is not a reliable warning signal, since you can lose two to three litres of fluid before you feel thirsty. And once you feel the early symptoms of heat exhaustion — dizziness or muscle cramps — your body temperature has already begun to rise. Chills and confusion may ensue. You should stop exercising and take fluids at once; otherwise you may suffer heat stroke.

When heat stroke sets in, body temperature soars. The skin becomes red and hot, and sweating may stop. A fever of 41 degrees Celsius or higher — even for a short period — can damage the brain and other organs. Heat stroke can be fatal if the victim's temperature is not brought under control quickly by immersing him in cold water or by other means.

In order to avoid heat injury, you should drink plenty of fluids before, during and after you exercise. Plain cool water is best, as explained on pages 125-127. You should ease up on exercise in hot, humid weather. High humidity slows the evaporation of perspiration from your skin. As a result, you will perspire more heavily, but the perspiration will be less effective as a coolant than it is in drier conditions.

Cold-related injuries are less problematic than injuries from heat, since you can maintain or boost your body temperature just by exercising harder and putting on more clothes. The most common injury arising from cold is frostbite — the freezing of tissue in subfreezing temperatures.

Dull, white, numbed patches of skin indicate the initial stages of frostbite, during which ice crystals form within the fluid of cells and tissues. Hands, feet, ears and the face are the most vulnerable. Prompt, but gradual, rewarming of the affected area will usually prevent any damage. Once normal skin colour and sensitivity return, the victim should seek medical care.

Hypothermia is a more insidious injury. The body conserves heat in cold weather by cutting off circulation to the hands and feet and by shivering. If the person at risk remains outdoors, body temperature falls and the first telltale signs of hypothermia — drowsiness, confusion, clumsiness and muscle weakness — may appear. Shivering may cease, and unconsciousness may follow. When body temperature drops rapidly, physical collapse, or even death, can result.

To minimize danger from cold, take the following precautions:

Avoid fatigue, which is the true cause of most hypothermia. If you conserve your energy, exercise will keep you warm.

Dress in layers. Trapped air is a far better insulator than any cloth, no matter how thick. Several layers of light clothing will trap air well, and are easy to remove as you warm up.

Stay dry. Wet clothing conducts heat away from your body far more quickly than dry clothing does.

Wear a cap. Because your head is the body's biggest radiator of heat, a cap can prevent heat loss.

Conditioning Your Stress Points

Most sports and related activities have particular injuries that are prevalent among their participants. There are some exceptions: tennis elbow is a form of tendinitis that you can get not only from playing tennis, but also from gardening, carpentry and other activities that involve repetitive forceful arm and wrist movements. Most sports do, however, have their own set of stress points. For example, the legs provide the main propulsive force in both cycling and running, but cyclists often complain of strained muscles in the neck and hamstrings, while runners tend to have the most problems in the knee, shin and lower back. Other sporting activities stress entirely different parts of the body: stop-and-start sports such as tennis jeopardize the ankles, whereas swimming may lead to shoulder pain.

While injuries are not always preventable, it is possible to reduce your chances of getting hurt by identifying your high-stress points and conditioning those parts of your body. Many cases of runner's knee, for instance, can be prevented by a good strengthening and stretching programme for the quadriceps muscles along the front of your thigh.

The chart opposite indicates the major points of stress for many common activities and cites the pages in this book where you can find routines to strengthen and stretch those parts of the body. Make use of these techniques to protect yourself against potential injury. Or, if you are recovering from injury, you can use the same routines to help speed the healing process. As a rule of thumb, you can generally exercise an injured body part provided that you feel no pain. If you do feel pain, reduce the intensity of your exercise or discontinue it altogether. You should consult a sports-medicine specialist or other doctor if the pain becomes severe or if you suffer recurring or persistent pain.

Sport-by-Sport Injury Guide

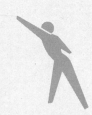

AEROBIC DANCE
pages 44-59, 68-91, 116-119

Aerobic dance can result in shin splints and other lower leg and knee injuries. Be sure to wear appropriate aerobic dance shoes and to perform low-impact routines that keep at least one foot on the floor at all times.

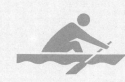

ROWING
pages 72-77, 100-117

Rowing is a powerful aerobic and muscular conditioner, and rowers enjoy a remarkably low injury rate. Nevertheless, rowers — particularly novices — often experience muscle soreness in their quadriceps, shoulders and upper arms, and can especially benefit from shoulder-stretching exercises.

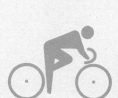

CYCLING
pages 46-47, 68-77, 100-103, 122-123

Although cycling involves no pounding, injuries are not uncommon, particularly among distance cyclists. Aches and pains include tendinitis in the ankle and knee, wrist strain, sore quadriceps and a sore neck. Be sure to wear the proper riding gear and use pedals with toe clips.

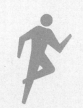

RUNNING
pages 44-59, 68-91, 116-119

Stress injuries to runners' knees, lower legs and feet are common. Runners also suffer from lower back pain. Especially important are good running shoes and proper posture. Runners should stretch their calf muscles frequently. Those with knee problems should strengthen the quadriceps muscles along the front of the thighs.

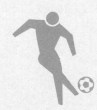

FOOTBALL
pages 46-59, 68-91

Strength and endurance are important ingredients for football. A good stretching and strengthening programme can be most effective in reducing both hamstring and calf muscle pulls, knee pain and ankle sprains.

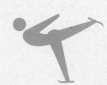

SKATING
pages 44-59, 72-77

Both ice and roller skating are strenuous activities that can result in stress injuries of the lower extremities. Skaters are prone to ankle injuries, tendinitis, shin splints and knee pain. Be sure to condition the quadriceps and ankle muscles.

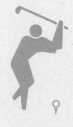

GOLF
pages 108-123

Golf can be a relaxing activity, but the forceful body rotation and momentum caused by swinging the golf club can place stress on the shoulders, spine and neck. Pay special attention to flexibility exercises for the shoulders and back.

SKIING
pages 104-119

Cross-country skiers are less likely to suffer acute injury, but forceful poling may strain their upper arms and lower back. Downhill skiers are far more prone to acute injuries as a result of falls than they are to stress injuries.

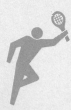

RACKET SPORTS
pages 46-59, 100-121

Tennis, racketball and squash frequently cause stress injuries to the forearm, shoulder and neck. The stop-and-start action can also strain the ankle and lower leg. Wear the proper shoes and pay special attention to good technique, particularly for the backhand strokes, which can cause tennis elbow if they are performed incorrectly.

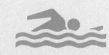

SWIMMING
pages 108-123

Of all sports, swimming is among the least stressful. However, because swimming uses full shoulder rotations and frequent head turning, the shoulders and neck can become injured and should be properly conditioned.

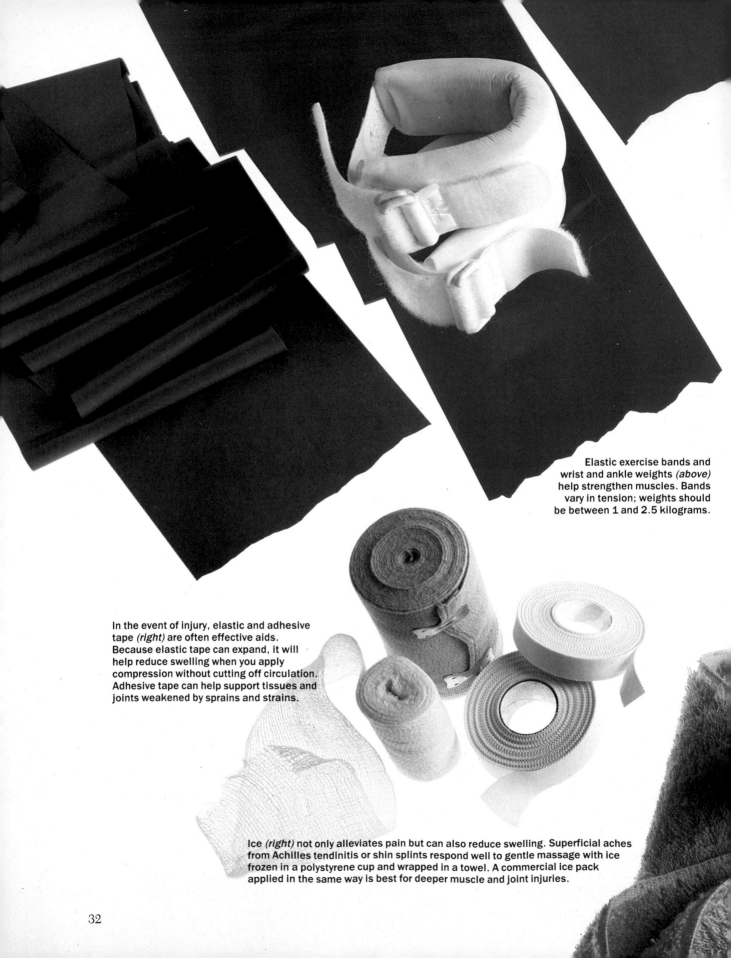

Elastic exercise bands and wrist and ankle weights *(above)* help strengthen muscles. Bands vary in tension; weights should be between 1 and 2.5 kilograms.

In the event of injury, elastic and adhesive tape *(right)* are often effective aids. Because elastic tape can expand, it will help reduce swelling when you apply compression without cutting off circulation. Adhesive tape can help support tissues and joints weakened by sprains and strains.

Ice *(right)* not only alleviates pain but can also reduce swelling. Superficial aches from Achilles tendinitis or shin splints respond well to gentle massage with ice frozen in a polystyrene cup and wrapped in a towel. A commercial ice pack applied in the same way is best for deeper muscle and joint injuries.

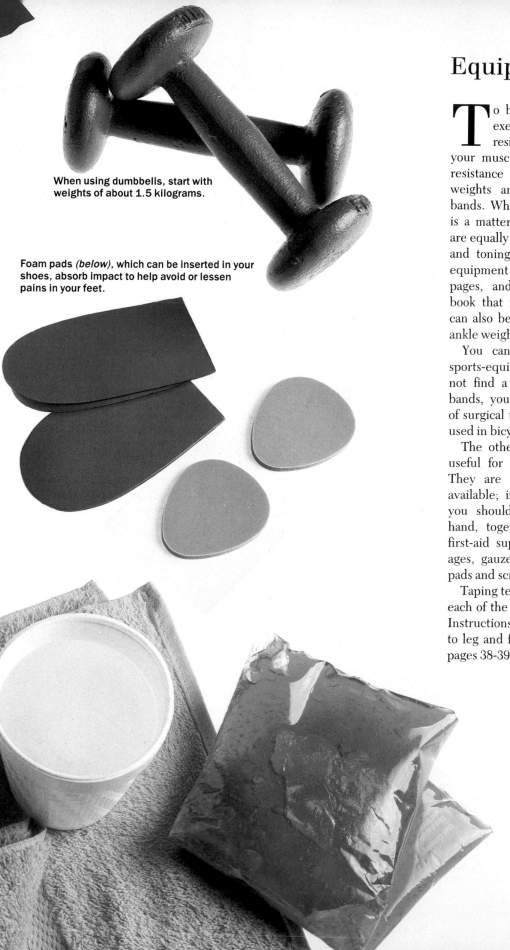

When using dumbbells, start with weights of about 1.5 kilograms.

Foam pads *(below)*, which can be inserted in your shoes, absorb impact to help avoid or lessen pains in your feet.

Equipment

To be effective, many of the exercises in this book require resistance to the movement of your muscles. You can supply this resistance in two ways — with weights and with elastic exercise bands. Which technique you choose is a matter of convenience, as they are equally effective in strengthening and toning muscles. Both types of equipment are shown on these two pages, and every exercise in this book that is performed with bands can also be performed with hand or ankle weights.

You can buy weights at many sports-equipment shops. If you cannot find a shop that sells exercise bands, you can make your own out of surgical tubing or the inner tubes used in bicycle tyres.

The other items shown here are useful for easing aches and pains. They are inexpensive and readily available; if you exercise regularly, you should always have them on hand, together with such standard first-aid supplies as adhesive bandages, gauze bandages, sterile gauze pads and scissors.

Taping techniques are explained in each of the following three chapters. Instructions on applying ice massage to leg and foot injuries are given on pages 38-39 and 64-65.

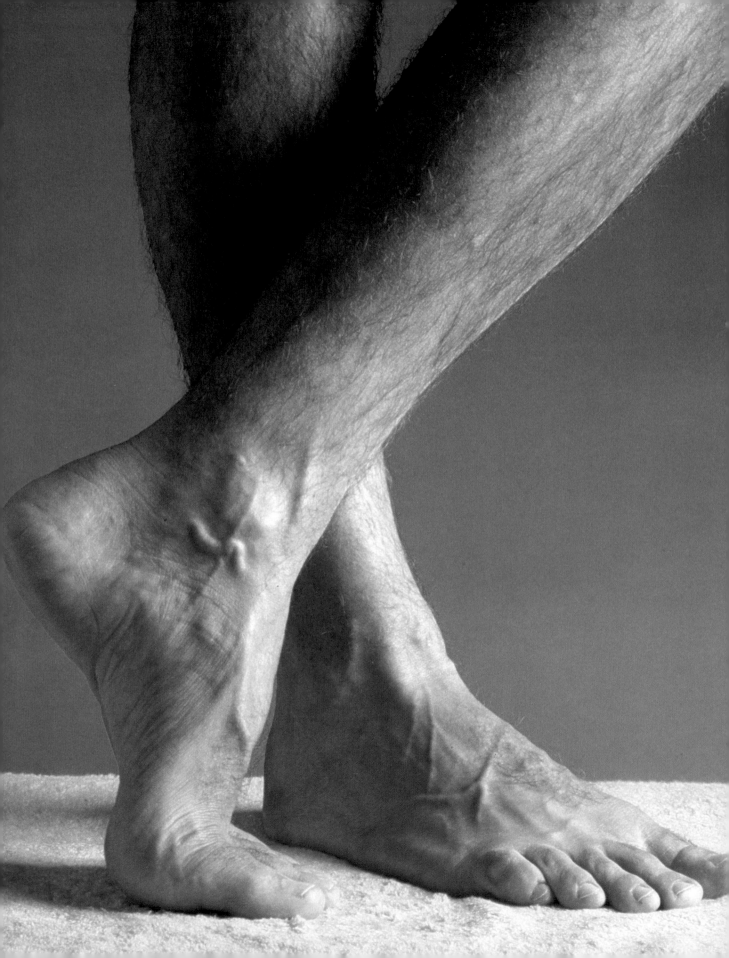

CHAPTER TWO

The Lower Leg

*The major site of impact — and
injury — during exercise*

More athletic and sports-related injuries occur in the lower leg — including the ankle and foot — than in any other region of the body. Because it absorbs the cumulative impact of walking, running, jumping, kicking and dancing, the lower leg is subject to problems ranging from blisters to stress fractures. According to a survey of more than 8,000 people treated at a San Francisco sports-medicine clinic over a five-year period, running caused the most injuries, and more than 40 per cent of all running injuries occurred below the knee. Of course, you do not have to be a runner to sustain a lower leg injury — almost any active person is susceptible. In the same sports-medicine study, more than 36 per cent of all basketball injuries affected the lower leg, as did 21 per cent of injuries linked to tennis. Aerobic dancers, skiers and soccer players also injure their feet, ankles and lower legs.

You can think of the calf, ankle and foot as a single biomechanical unit that forms a lever whose functions are essential to the performance of just about every locomotive activity. Although exceedingly complex in structure and function, this lever's basic components are the calf muscles, the Achilles tendon, the heel bone and the plantar fascia, which runs from the heel bone to the toes. These structures are interconnected, forming a sling that runs from under your knee to your heel and then along the bottom of your foot to your toes. To stand on your toes, for instance, your calf muscles must do most of the work. When you contract your calf muscles, your Achilles tendon lifts your heel bone, which in turn pulls on your plantar fascia.

The calf muscles, which flex the ankle and point the foot, are assisted and opposed by muscles that extend the ankle and draw the toes and forefoot up. These muscles are located on the anterior, or front, of the leg, opposite the calf muscles, and run between the tibia and fibula, the bones of the lower leg. The tendons that attach these muscles to your forefoot run along the front of your ankle. If you turn your toes up, you can feel these tendons tighten along the top of your foot and the base of your shinbone. Chronically tight calf muscles will cause an imbalance in the musculature of the leg, pulling on the heel bone and making the foot extend downwards; the opposing muscles will then tighten in order to hold the foot in a normal position. This tightening can cause a number of problems, including anterior muscle pain, commonly known as shin splints; Achilles tendinitis, which is inflammation of the Achilles tendon below the calf; tenderness along the bottom of the foot, which is known as plantar fasciitis; and stress fractures of the metatarsal bones.

Tight calf muscles are usually a consequence of weakness, overtraining or a combination of the two. If you work a weak muscle too hard, it will tighten up. That is why you may feel stiff the morning after a particularly rigorous tennis game. But if you increase your fitness level gradually, rather than try to make up for a week of inactivity with a gruelling exercise session, your muscles will adapt rather than become fatigued and tight.

In addition to injuries that stem from muscle fatigue, the lower leg and foot can become injured by such acute traumas as twisting your ankle or stubbing your toe. Stop-and-start sports such as tennis and basketball place the greatest stress on the lower leg, and muscle pulls and tendon tears are frequent as a result.

Many experts agree that ankle injuries, particularly those on the outside of the ankle, are the most frequent lower leg problems. But considering the stress so many sports put on the ankle, it is amazing that the ankle is not injured even more often than it is. A single anklebone, the talus, must support the weight of your entire body apart from your foot, and frequently — when you run or jump, for instance — it supports several times as much weight.

Some ankle and calf injuries can be avoided simply by wearing the appropriate shoes. If you play stop-and-start games in running shoes, for example, you may be courting trouble, since these shoes provide neither ankle nor lateral support. Old shoes can also place undue stress

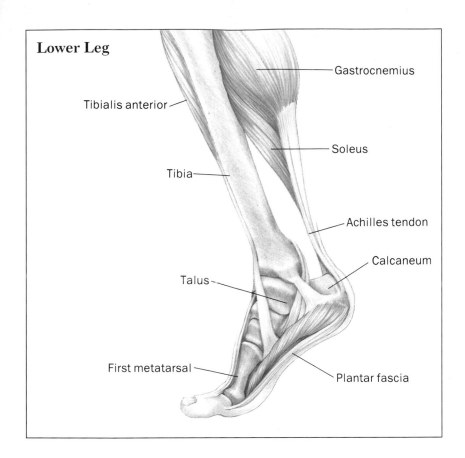

Lower Leg

Tibialis anterior

Gastrocnemius

Soleus

Tibia

Achilles tendon

Calcaneum

Talus

First metatarsal

Plantar fascia

on the ankle, particularly if the outside part of the heel is worn down.

Maintaining muscular balance can help to prevent injury. An activity such as running will strengthen and tighten the calf muscles, for instance, at the expense of the opposing shin muscles. Therefore, if you run regularly, you should be sure to stretch your calf muscles and strengthen your shin muscles.

Stretching calf muscles can also contribute to keeping your Achilles tendon flexible and less vulnerable to injury. Also make sure that the midsoles of your shoes provide enough cushioning and that your heels are comfortably but firmly held in place.

Even with proper conditioning, overexertion or mishaps may offset your best efforts to remain injury-free. If you do suffer a stress injury, the following two pages explain how to give yourself an ice massage, one of the most effective first-aid techniques. The remainder of this chapter demonstrates taping techniques to support injured body parts and to help prevent reinjury, as well as exercises to help hasten your rehabilitation and keep you in good condition once you are able to return to a full schedule of activities.

Ice Massage

Almost all athletic soft-tissue aches and injuries — soreness, sprains, strains, muscle spasms — respond to ice massage. Icing will reduce pain, slow down bleeding and restrict swelling as well as speed recovery. Since the massage technique involves moving the ice constantly, there is little chance of damaging your skin.

Ice alleviates pain by reducing muscle spasm in the injured area and inhibiting nerve impulses. But the principal benefit of icing is to help stop internal bleeding by causing injured capillaries to contract. The more these capillaries contract, the less blood can collect around injured tissues. Preventing blood from collecting in these areas minimizes any swelling and discomfort, and also shortens the recovery time. The sooner you can move the injured area, the less you will need to be concerned about muscle atrophy and loss of strength, which in many cases lead to reinjury.

Unless a doctor specifically instructs you to do so, never apply heat to a swollen area. Heat will dilate the capillaries and increase swelling.

One way you can apply ice to the injured area is to crush ice cubes, wrap the ice in a towel and press the cold pack on the injured area. The towel prevents direct contact between the ice and your skin, and thus saves your skin from chance of damage. Another way to ice many injuries is through ice massage, an effective form of icing that involves rubbing the ice directly on the tender area. Ice cups — polystyrene or paper cups filled with water and then frozen — are a handy means of applying ice massage, and if you tend to be prone to minor injuries or can anticipate occasional bouts of low-level shin splints or Achilles tendinitis, you should keep several of these cups stored in your freezer. The ice-filled cup enables you to hold the ice firmly and apply it directly to the site of your injury without chilling your fingers. Whenever possible, raise the injured area to hip level or higher to help restrict blood flow and further reduce swelling. Then rub the skin with circular or back-and-forth movements. As the ice melts, peel away a strip of the cup to expose more ice.

Perform an ice massage for 10 to 15 minutes at a time. Stop the ice massage if your skin begins to turn red or if you experience a burning sensation. Repeat three or four times a day or as often as you can until the swelling is reduced.

Elevate the injured limb and place it on a towel. Place the ice cup over the injured area and press firmly. For most injuries, such as those of the ankle *(opposite)*, massage in a circular motion with the ice cup. For Achilles tendinitis *(inset)*, rub the ice up and down from the calf to the heel.

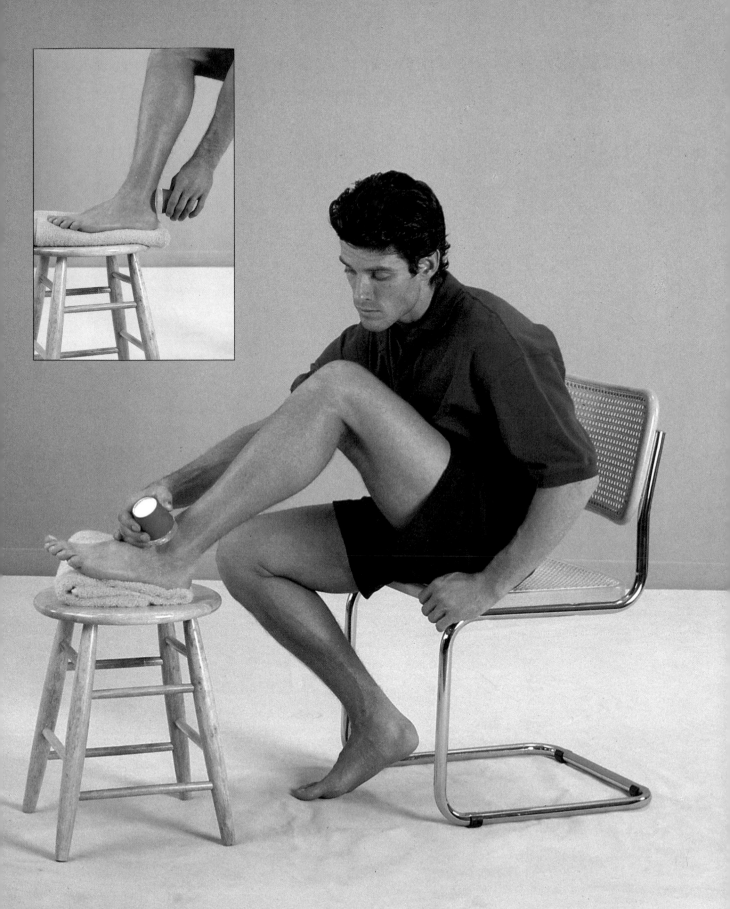

Taping/1

Many coaches and athletes believe that taping — a technique commonly used to treat injuries of the muscles, tendons and ligaments — is valuable in aiding recovery from sports-related injuries. Because such injuries can take a long time to heal, the muscles and support tissue round an injury site may lose some strength and mobility. As a result, you are vulnerable to reinjury when you return to your full schedule of activities. If you apply some form of support, such as adhesive taping, you may alleviate stress and lessen the risk of reinjury.

All taping for support — even that which is done by a professional — causes some restriction in function, but good taping techniques can minimize this problem.

Use tape that is 4 to 5 centimetres wide; the perforated variety can be torn into strips easily. Wash your skin and shave your body hair wherever you apply tape directly to the skin. If the adhesive irritates your skin, remove the tape and apply a protective wrapping of gauze before taping again. You should also use gauze if you are taping a large area that you do not wish to shave or if you are allergic to the adhesive.

Only a doctor or sports-medicine specialist should apply tape to a serious injury such as a fractured foot or ankle, since overly tight taping can impede circulation and cause other problems. Also, only a doctor can properly assess the extent of damage in an acute injury; applying tape yourself may mask symptoms and delay proper treatment. Proper taping does take practice to be effective in reducing the risk of injury; furthermore, a bad taping technique or poorly applied taping may accentuate the risk of injury. But you can safely tape many mild strains and sprains such as Grade I ankle sprains, described on page 46.

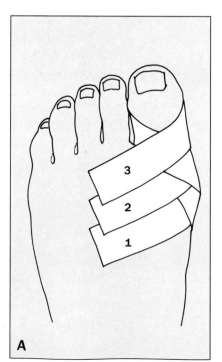 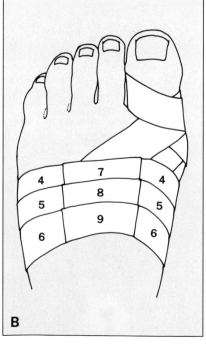

A: To support the big toe, start the first strip of tape underneath the ball of the foot, wrap it up the side and then loop it round the big toe, ending on top of the foot to form half a figure-of-eight. Do the same with two more overlapping strips of tape. *B:* Secure the toe wrap by using three tie-down strips (4, 5 and 6) round the foot. Apply three short strips (7, 8 and 9) on the top of the foot to fasten the ends of the tape. (Tape adheres better to tape than to skin.)

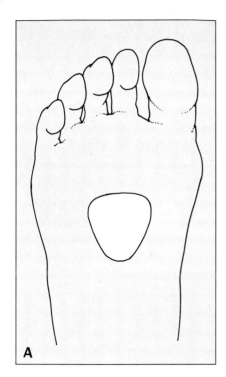

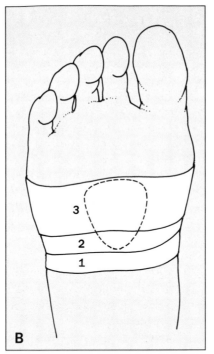

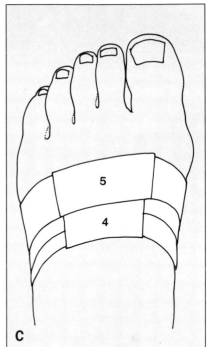

A: To support the metatarsal arch, place an oval foam footpad where support is most needed. *B:* Secure the pad with three strips of tape, leaving a gap between the ends of the tape on the top of the foot. *C:* Apply two short strips on the top of the foot to fasten the ends of the tape.

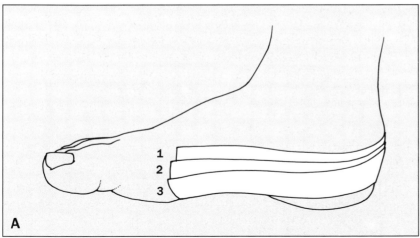

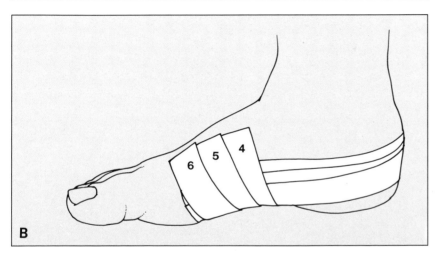

A: To help ease excessive pronation and pain along the bottom of the foot, keep the foot in a neutral position and apply three strips of overlapping tape from the outside of the foot, round the heel and ending near the ball of the foot. *B:* Tie the strips down with three overlapping strips that are perpendicular to the layer below.

Taping/2

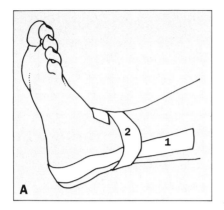

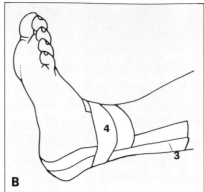

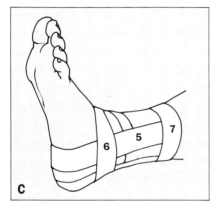

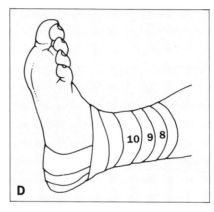

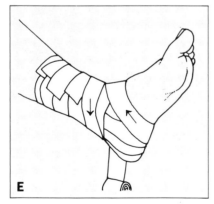

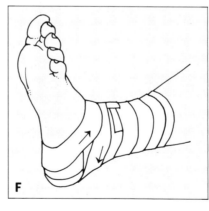

A: To tape your ankle for a mild sprain, hold your foot at a right angle to your leg. Place strip 1 about 10 centimetres above the inside ankle, carry it under the heel and end it about 10 centimetres above the outside ankle just below the calf. Encircle the leg just above the ankle with strip 2. *B:* Begin strip 3 on the inside of the leg and overlap strip 1 by about 2 centimetres. Overlap strip 2 with strip 4. *C:* Follow the same overlapping procedure with strips 5 and 6. Encircle the leg with strip 7 and anchor the tops of the straps. *D:* Work down the leg with overlapping strips 8, 9 and 10. *E:* Lock the heel in place by wrapping tape round the heel and ankle as shown. *F:* Continue the ankle taping, being careful not to leave any gaps that may allow pinching or a blister, especially along the Achilles tendon.

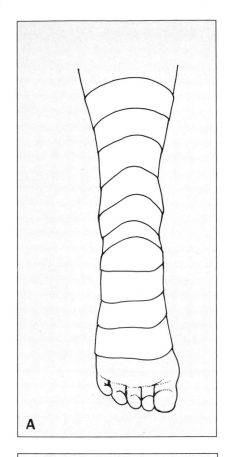

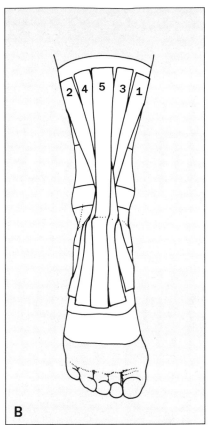

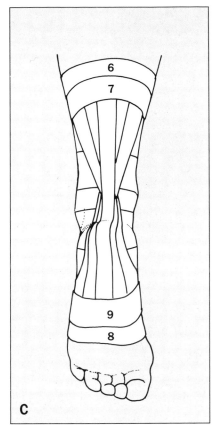

A: To begin taping for Achilles tendinitis or calf muscle strain, keep the foot at a right angle to the leg and apply an underwrap, anchoring it with tape at midcalf and midfoot. *B:* Apply a fan over the underwrap using five strips of tape running from the foot to the calf. *C:* Tie the fan down with strip 6, which encircles the calf. Overlap with strip 7. Secure the other end of the fan with strips 8 and 9.

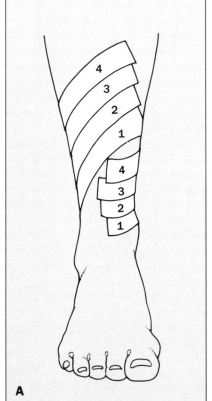

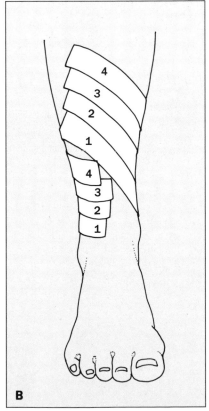

A: For shin splint pain along the outer front of the leg, begin the first strip of tape just above the inside ankle joint. Wrap the tape round the back of the leg and spiral upwards, finishing on the inside front of the leg as shown. Overlap more strips of tape, applying as many as needed. *B:* For shin splint pain on the inner side of the leg, use the same technique but start the tape just above the outside ankle.

Foot

The foot is an elastic arch in which muscles, tendons and ligaments provide support. This arch flattens somewhat as your body weight bears down on it, and when it flattens, it stores energy in much the same way as a rubber ball stores energy when you bounce it. This energy is released as you take a step, adding "bounce" to your stride. Without this bounce, your muscles would require twice as much oxygen for the same amount of work.

A connective tissue called the plantar fascia runs along the bottom of your foot between your heel bone and the base of your toes. It constantly absorbs stresses, especially when you run. Plantar fasciitis — a tear in this tissue — is characterized by pain and swelling under the heel. A frequent runner's complaint, it is often associated with heel spurs, painful calcification of the point where the plantar fascia attaches to the heel bone. Plantar fasciitis and heel spurs are often caused by excessive foot pronation, inadequate arch support and stiff shoes.

You can treat heel spurs and plantar fasciitis with ice massage. Another way to help alleviate these conditions, is to place a doughnut or horseshoe-shaped cushioning pad in the heel of your shoe.

If you are prone to foot injuries, you should engage in a programme of strengthening and stretching. Perform the exercises shown on these two pages at least twice a day.

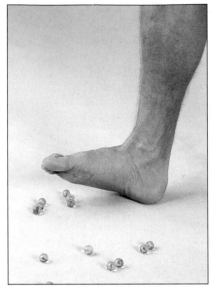

Place about a dozen marbles on the floor. Pick them up one by one with your toes, placing them in a group about 15 centimetres away.

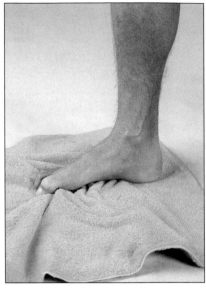

Cover a bare floor with a towel and place your foot at one end, pointing your toes towards the far end. Grip the towel with your toes and pull the far end towards you. To increase the effort, place a 1 kilogram weight at the end of the towel.

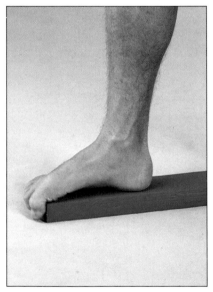

Place a board on the floor and step on it, letting your toes extend over the end. Curl your toes, gripping the wood. Hold for five seconds and relax. Do 10 repetitions.

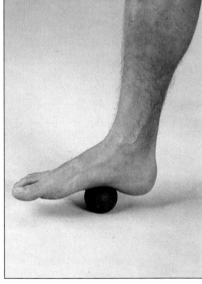

Gently massage and relax the muscles and tendons on the underside of your foot by placing a small ball on the floor and rolling your foot over it.

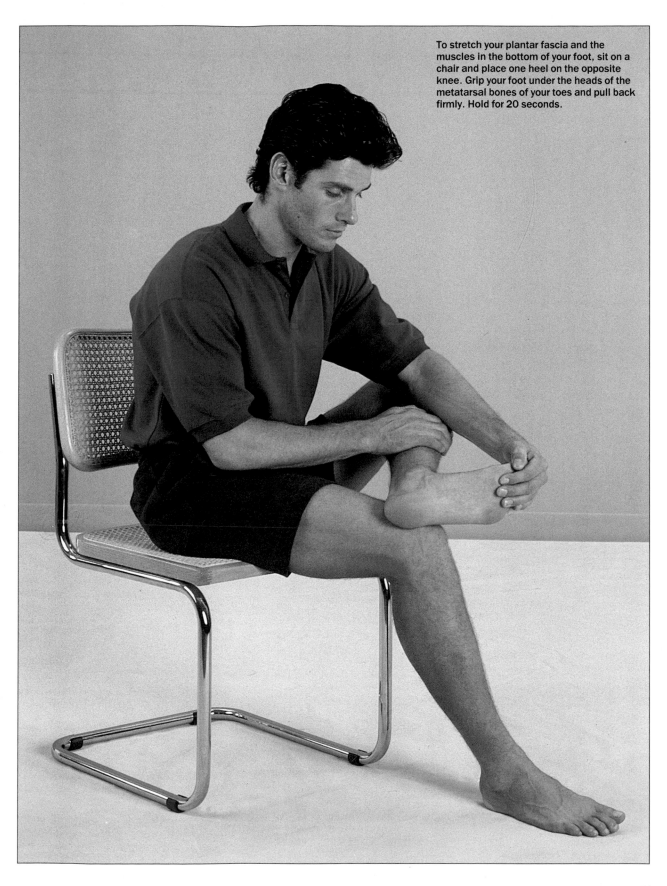

To stretch your plantar fascia and the muscles in the bottom of your foot, sit on a chair and place one heel on the opposite knee. Grip your foot under the heads of the metatarsal bones of your toes and pull back firmly. Hold for 20 seconds.

Ankle/1

Although the ankle may appear to be delicate and unstable, it is quite durable, particularly for such a small joint that bears a great deal of weight. The ligaments and tendons that hold the ankle together are some of the strongest in your body. The weakest part of the joint is its musculature, which does not stabilize it as well as the musculature in other joints.

An ankle sprain is a partial or complete rupture of one or more of the ligaments connecting the bones of the joint. Of all sports injuries, ankle sprains are the most common: in a study at West Point Military Academy in the United States, about one third of all cadets who participated in sports sustained an ankle sprain. Similarly, a study of 3,000 secondary school athletes showed that a significant percentage of their sports-related injuries were those of the ankle. Of these, sprains were by far the most common.

Ankle injuries are classified into one of three categories: Grade I, in which there is minimal pain and swelling, and you are able to walk without impairment; Grade II, in which there is moderate pain and swelling, and you have difficulty standing and walking; and Grade III, in which there is severe pain and swelling, and you are unable to move the ankle much or put weight on it. Grade III injuries require the immediate attention of a doctor or a hospital emergency room. While not as serious, Grade II injuries also require medical attention from a general practitioner or sports-medicine specialist. The best treatment for Grade I ankle sprain is RICE, which is explained on pages 24-25.

Begin exercising your ankle as soon as possible after your injury: as long as you are not in any pain, you are not harming your ankle. Start by walking slowly, and gradually take longer and faster strides. Stationary cycling is also a good way in which to recondition your ankle.

The best way to stabilize the joint and avoid injuring it again is to strengthen the muscles in your lower leg; this approach is also a good preventive measure if you have not sustained an ankle injury. The exercises demonstrated on this and the next five pages will provide overall conditioning benefits for the ankle.

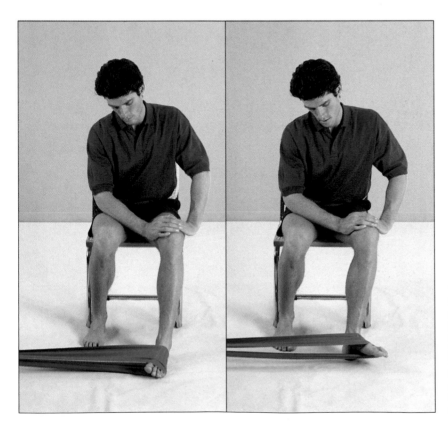

To strengthen the ankle eversion muscles, which turn your foot outwards, attach an elastic exercise band to a piece of stable furniture such as a table leg. Sit on a chair so that your right side is nearer the table leg, and loop the band snugly round your left foot *(far left)*. Keep your heel and knee still, but turn your foot up and out to the left as far as you can *(left)*. Perform three sets of 10 repetitions. Then turn your chair round and repeat for the right foot.

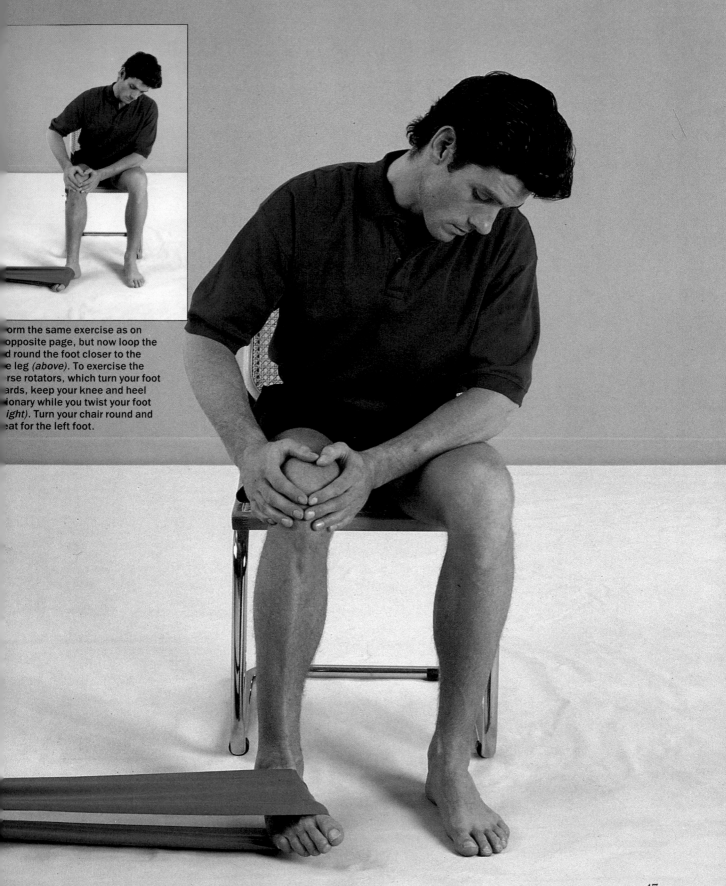

orm the same exercise as on
opposite page, but now loop the
d round the foot closer to the
e leg *(above)*. To exercise the
rse rotators, which turn your foot
ards, keep your knee and heel
onary while you twist your foot
ight). Turn your chair round and
at for the left foot.

47

Ankle/2

To perform alternative rotation exercises for the ankle, attach the elastic band to a table leg and sit on the floor with your knees bent at a right angle. Loop the band round your far foot for eversion rotation exercises *(right)*, and your near foot for inversion rotations. If you do not have an exercise band, lie on your right side on a bench or firm bed with your left foot extended over the end. Attach an ankle weight to your foot and perform eversion rotations by turning your foot up *(below)*. Turn over and repeat the exercises for your right foot.

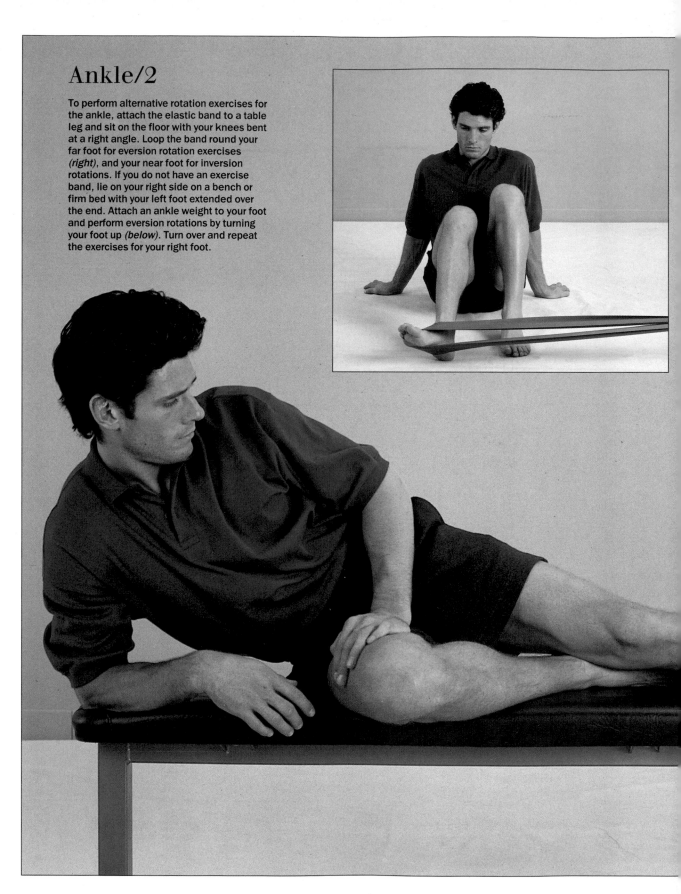

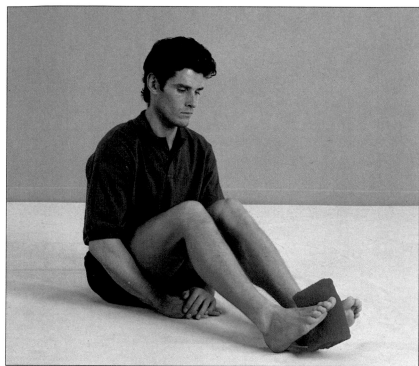

To perform inversion rotation exercises without an elastic exercise band, sit on the floor with your knees bent so that your upper and lower legs form a right angle. Place a towel between your feet and press them together as hard as you can for five seconds, then relax.

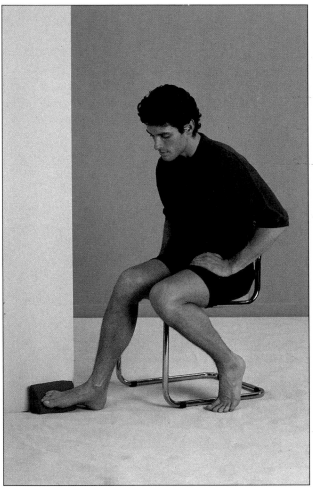

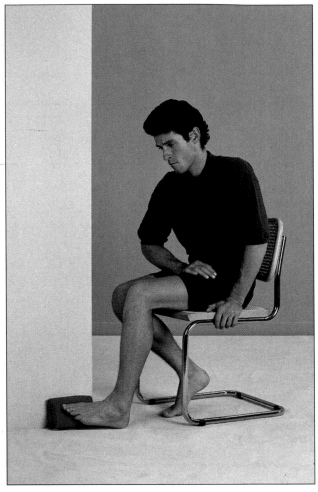

To perform eversion ankle rotations while seated, place your chair near the corner of a wall or the leg of a desk so that your right forefoot rests against it. Put a towel between your foot and the wall. Keep your heel on the floor and press the outside of your foot against the wall as hard as you can for five seconds, then relax. Perform three sets of 10 repetitions. Turn your chair and repeat for your left foot.

To strengthen the inversion rotators using isometrics, place your chair next to the corner of a wall or the leg of a desk. Put a towel next to the wall to serve as a cushion. Keep your heel in one place and press the inside of your left foot against the towel for five seconds, then relax. Perform three sets of 10 repetitions. Turn your chair round and repeat for your right foot.

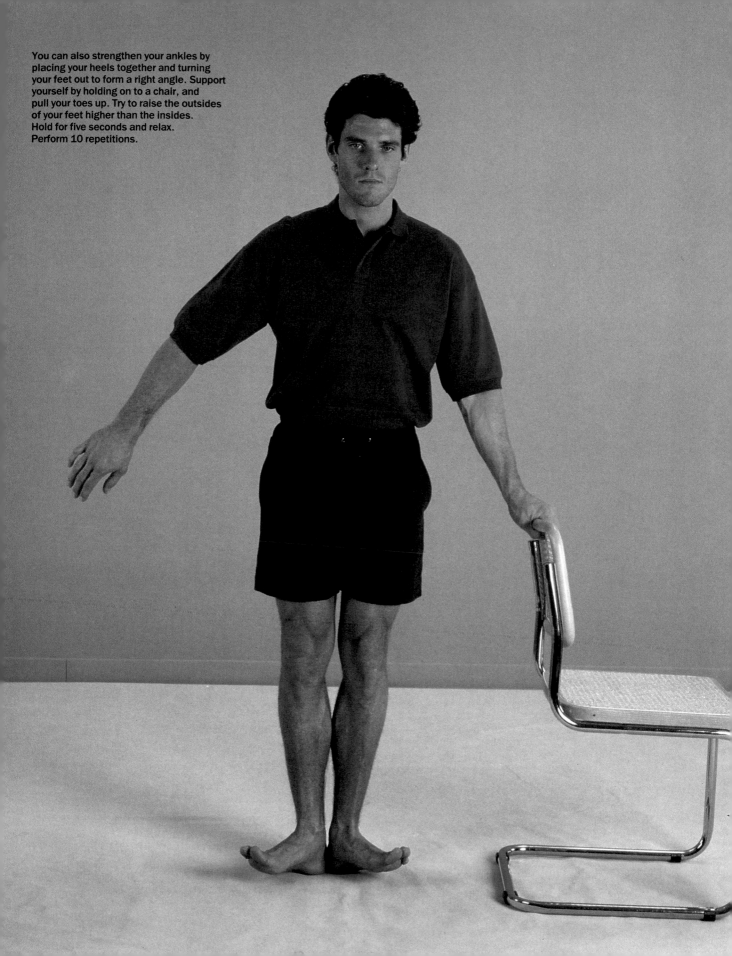

You can also strengthen your ankles by placing your heels together and turning your feet out to form a right angle. Support yourself by holding on to a chair, and pull your toes up. Try to raise the outsides of your feet higher than the insides. Hold for five seconds and relax. Perform 10 repetitions.

Calf and Achilles Tendon/1

The major calf muscle, the gastrocnemius, passes behind the knee and attaches to the Achilles tendon, which is anchored behind the ankle in the heel bone. Because it is a two-joint muscle, the gastrocnemius has twice the chance of being overstretched, strained or torn as a one-joint muscle. When you lunge to make a difficult tennis shot, for example, both knee and ankle are extended, and you may strain the gastrocnemius. Your calf will feel sore and the muscle may go into spasm, a sudden, involuntary muscle contraction that can produce intense pain. When this occurs, perform calf stretches immediately and massage with ice. Consult a doctor if the spasm continues.

The complaint of Achilles tendinitis, or soreness of the Achilles tendon, is most often caused by fatigued and tight calf muscles, including the gastrocnemius and the smaller soleus. The tension produces inflammation, which may lead to swelling of the surrounding tissue and, in severe cases, excruciating pain. Achilles tendinitis usually responds well to a treatment of rest, ice massage and stretching.

The exercises shown here and on the following three pages help guard against calf injuries as well as Achilles tendinitis.

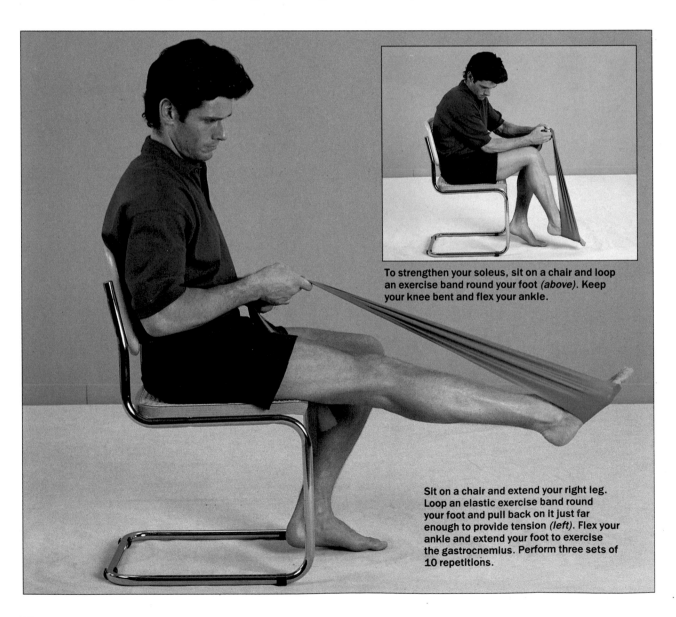

To strengthen your soleus, sit on a chair and loop an exercise band round your foot *(above)*. Keep your knee bent and flex your ankle.

Sit on a chair and extend your right leg. Loop an elastic exercise band round your foot and pull back on it just far enough to provide tension *(left)*. Flex your ankle and extend your foot to exercise the gastrocnemius. Perform three sets of 10 repetitions.

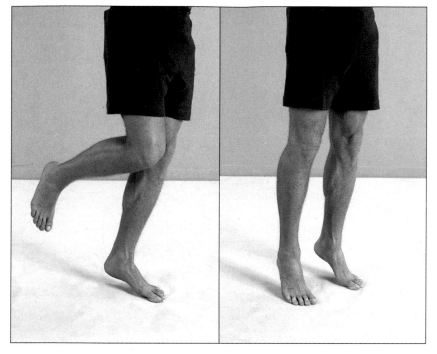

An effective strengthening technique known as eccentric contraction slowly lengthens the muscle as it reacts to an external force. Use this contraction to strengthen your calf muscles by rising up on your toes *(left)*. Lift your right foot off the floor and slowly lower your left heel back down *(far left)*. Repeat for your right leg.

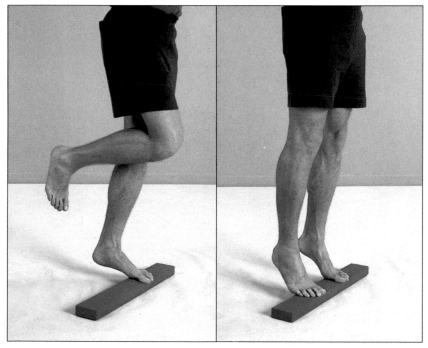

To increase the effort of the above exercise, place a wooden board on the floor. Stand on the board so that your heels extend over the edge. Rise up on your toes *(left)*. Lift your right foot off the board and slowly lower your left heel to the floor to perform an eccentric contraction of the left calf muscles *(far left)*. Repeat for your right calf.

Calf and Achilles Tendon/2

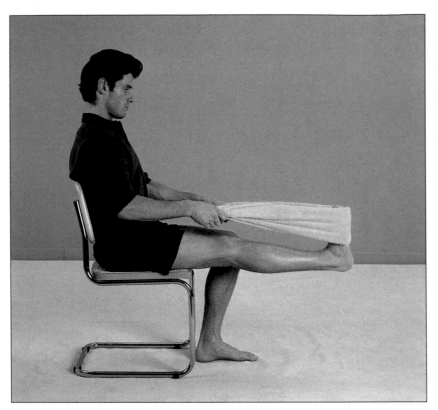

To stretch your gastrocnemius, sit on a chair and extend your right leg. Loop a towel over your foot and pull back until you feel your calf muscle extend. Hold for 20 seconds. Repeat at least once, then perform the same stretch on your left leg.

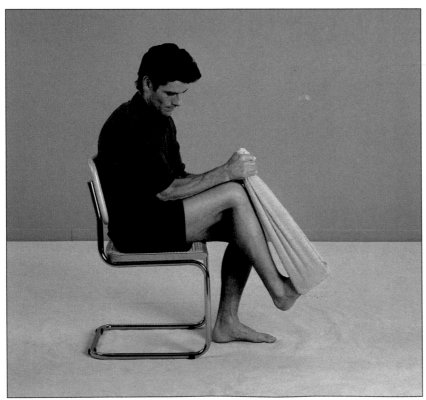

To stretch your soleus, sit on a chair and loop a towel under your right foot. Keep your knee bent and pull back on the towel until you feel a stretch in your calf. Hold for 20 seconds and repeat at least once. Then repeat the stretch for your left leg.

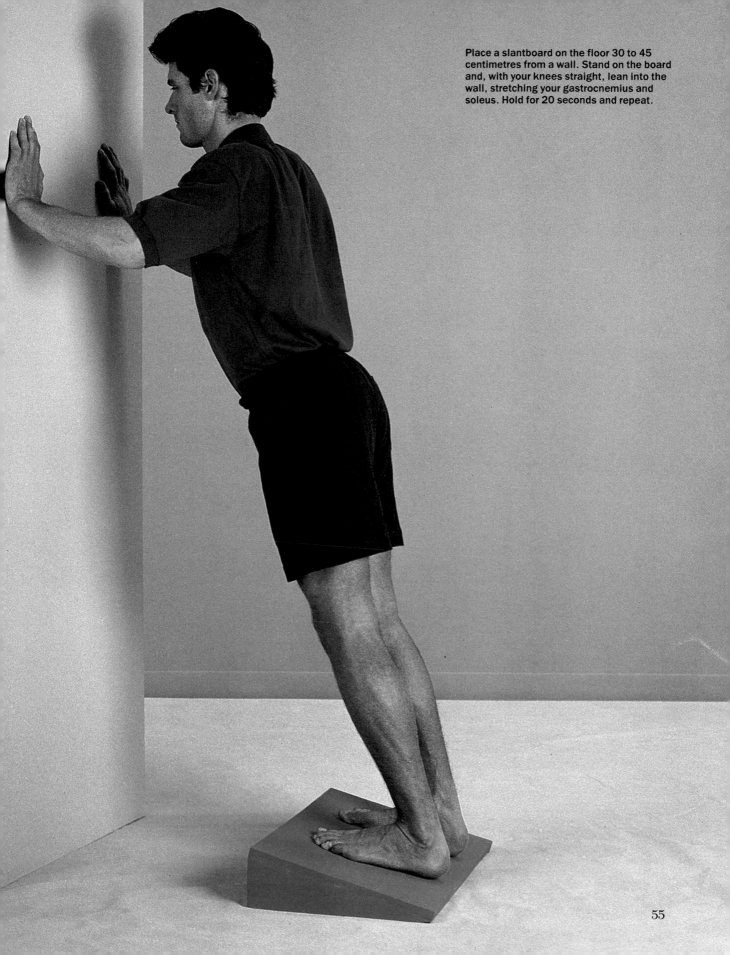

Place a slantboard on the floor 30 to 45 centimetres from a wall. Stand on the board and, with your knees straight, lean into the wall, stretching your gastrocnemius and soleus. Hold for 20 seconds and repeat.

Shin

The shin may appear bony and devoid of moving parts or major musculature, however, it sometimes causes active people a great deal of pain. Commonly referred to as shin splints, pain in the shin accounts for about 10 to 15 per cent of all running injuries. Actually, the term *shin splints* refers to a host of problems ranging in severity from mild tendinitis to stress fractures. Although shin splint sufferers rarely notice swelling, they often experience localized tenderness in the shin, and they usually feel pain on the front or the side of the leg after a workout, while walking or even when they are at rest.

Overtraining or inappropriate footwear can contribute to shin pain, but biomechanical problems may also be to blame, particularly excessive foot pronation, or inward rotation of the foot.

Shin splint pain will often subside if you reduce your level of exercise. Ice massage is also effective. Once the pain diminishes, you can begin an exercise programme that includes stretching the calf muscles *(pages 54-55)*, performing ankle inversion exercises *(pages 47-50)* and the exercises on these two pages. Chronic shin splints should be diagnosed and treated by a doctor.

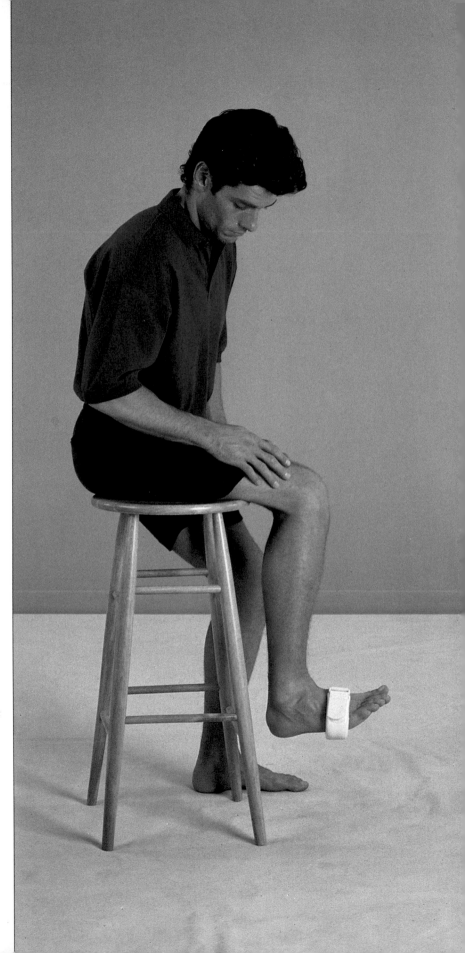

To strengthen your tibialis anterior, which is the major muscle in your shin, use a high stool and attach a 1.5 kilogram ankle weight to your right foot. With your left foot on the floor, half-sit on the stool and raise your right foot by flexing and extending the ankle. Perform three sets of 10 repetitions. Repeat for your left leg.

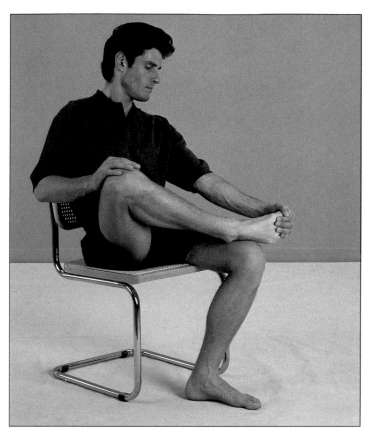

To stretch your right anterior tibial muscle while sitting on a chair, place your right ankle on your left knee and grasp the toes of your right foot with your left hand. Place your right hand on your right knee to stabilize the leg and pull back on your toes. Hold the stretch for at least 20 seconds. Repeat for your left leg.

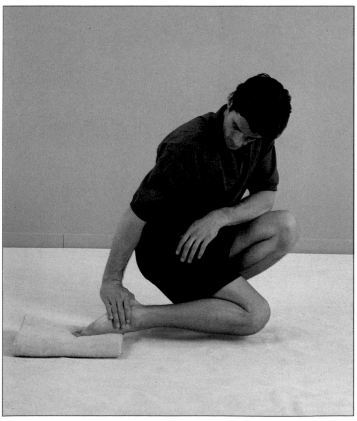

You can also stretch your anterior tibial muscles while sitting on the floor. Place a towel on the floor and, squatting on your left leg, kneel with your right so that the top of your right foot rests on the towel. Grasp your right heel with your right hand and lean back until you feel a stretch in your shin. Hold for at least 20 seconds, then repeat for the left leg.

Regaining Co-ordination

Even when you have fully reconditioned your muscles after an injury, you may still not have recovered all your co-ordination. When an injury forces you to rest, you inevitably lose some co-ordination between the central nervous system and the musculoskeletal system — the muscles, tendons, ligaments and joints. You must relearn this type of co-ordination, which is called proprioception.

Within your musculoskeletal system are specialized sensory organs that are called proprioceptors. These organs relay information about the positions of muscles and limbs to the central nervous system. Through these messages, the central nervous system keeps track of your movements. Proprioception permits you to perform many familiar and simple tasks, such as standing still without falling over, walking and running, without consciously thinking about your muscle movements. But injury may lead to the loss of a certain degree of proprioception, and in such cases muscle co-ordination will have to be relearned. Any loss of co-ordination can be especially noticeable when your lower leg is injured, since co-ordination among the tendons and muscles there is critical for all locomotion.

Proprioception training should begin as soon as you have regained muscle strength and flexibility. By performing a movement that uses various muscle groups, such as balancing on an unsteady board, you retrain nerves and muscles to synchronize movements. Your ultimate goal is to regain your sense of timing, balance and co-ordination.

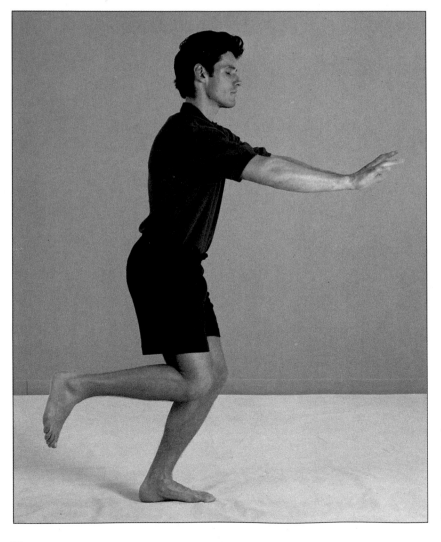

To improve co-ordination and balance after a lower leg or foot injury, stand up straight. Lift your uninjured foot off the floor and bend your knee so that your upper and lower leg form a right angle. Extend your arms in front of you and close your eyes. Bend your upright leg slightly and maintain this position for as long as you can.

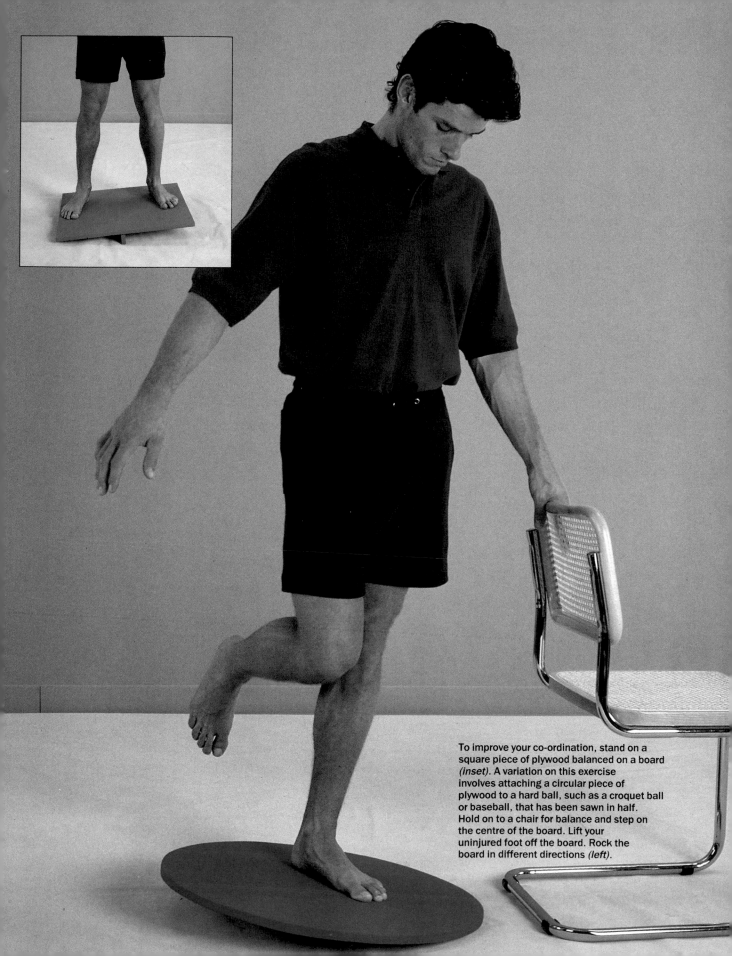

To improve your co-ordination, stand on a square piece of plywood balanced on a board *(inset)*. A variation on this exercise involves attaching a circular piece of plywood to a hard ball, such as a croquet ball or baseball, that has been sawn in half. Hold on to a chair for balance and step on the centre of the board. Lift your uninjured foot off the board. Rock the board in different directions *(left)*.

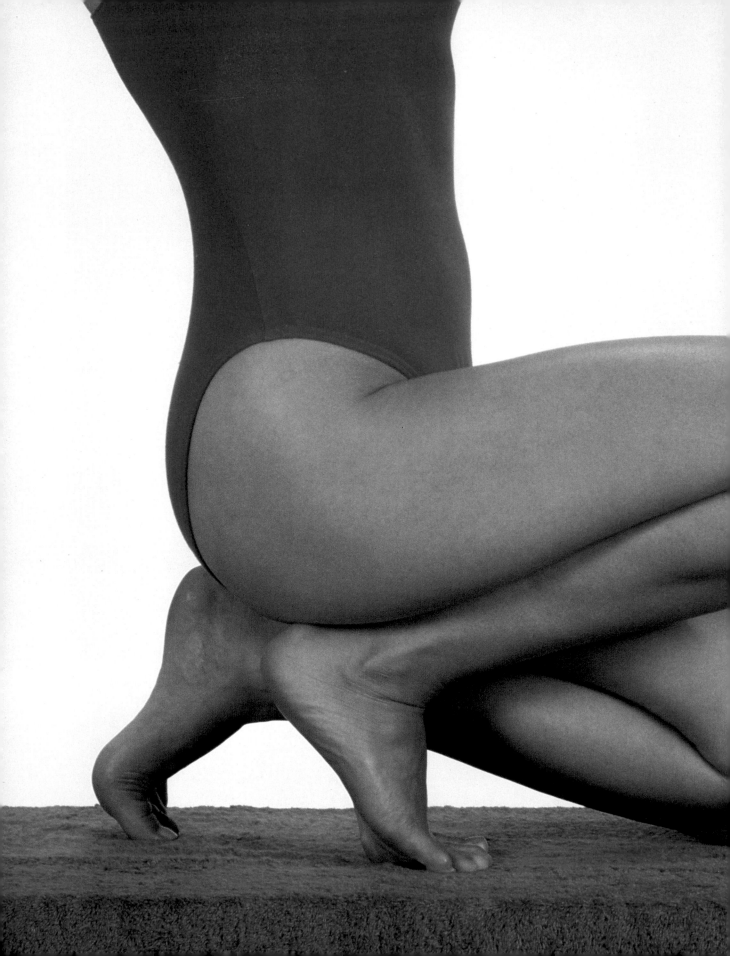

CHAPTER THREE

The Knee and Thigh

A range of problems and remedies for your largest joints and muscles

Almost anyone who is at all active — who runs, jumps, cycles, plays tennis, hikes or even climbs stairs regularly — can develop knee problems. In fact, considering the forces to which the knees are routinely subjected, it is not surprising that they are injured as frequently as they are. Knee problems account for one in four sports-related injuries, and three out of every four sports-related surgical repairs involve the knee. Even when you are doing something as commonplace as walking down a steep hill, your knees must be strong enough to withstand pressure amounting to three times your body weight. When you squat down, a part of each kneecap is subjected to pressures equivalent to several times your body weight.

People who are beginning an exercise programme or who intensify an existing routine are particularly prone to minor knee injuries, since flexing and extending the knee more than usual may cause minor swelling as a result of friction in the joint's components. Usually, the pain is caused by minor tendinitis, or inflammation of the tendons round the kneecap, and it will disappear after a day or two of rest. However, the likelihood of stress injuries to the knee and thigh can be significantly reduced by proper conditioning, which includes strengthening and stretching routines. While chronic or severe knee or thigh pain should be diagnosed and treated by a doctor, understanding the cause of your discomfort, along with a knowledge of the structure of the knee and thigh, may also help speed your recovery and prevent your injury from recurring.

At first glance, the knee appears to be unstable and awkwardly constructed. It is, however, one of the most secure joints in the body. The knee is supported by powerful ligaments contributing to an elaborate system of stays and pulleys that hold the joint together, extend and retract the lower leg and keep the kneecap from sliding off its track. The knees must also be able to bend and rotate, often simultaneously, and serve as shock absorbers for the upper body.

The muscles of the thigh — the quadriceps in front, which is usually the largest and most powerful muscle group of the body, and the hamstrings in the back — constitute the muscular support system for the knee. The quadriceps straighten the knee and extend the lower leg, while the hamstrings bend the knee and retract the lower leg. There are four other major groups of thigh muscles that attach to your pelvis and move your thigh: hip flexors raise your thigh; hip extensors draw your thigh backwards; adductors swing your leg inwards; and abductors pull your leg outwards. Some of the quadriceps and hamstring muscles are also included in these groups.

In addition to its other functions, the quadriceps muscle group guides and stabilizes the kneecap, or patella, as it glides over a U-shaped depression at the end of the thighbone. The kneecap increases the lever action of the quadriceps on the lower leg, substantially improving the power of this muscle group. Weak quadriceps muscles may lead to incorrect tracking of the kneecap in its groove. This, in turn, can cause diffuse pain under or round the kneecap, which is commonly known as runner's knee. This condition, more accurately called patellofemoral pain, accounts for approximately 60 per cent of all stress injuries to the knee. It commonly afflicts not only runners, but also cyclists, hikers and soccer players.

The next most common stress injuries to the knee are forms of tendinitis. This inflammation often occurs in the tendons connecting the quadriceps and the kneecap, and in those that attach the kneecap to the bone just below the knee. Tendinitis can be particularly troublesome since tendons have a relatively poor blood supply and may take a long time to heal if they are injured. Jumper's knee, tendinitis that occurs just below the kneecap, often troubles basketball players. Osgood-Schlatter disease, another type of tendinitis, results in a painful, swollen lump about 5 centimetres below the kneecap. A kind of "growing pain" of the knee seen most often in youngsters

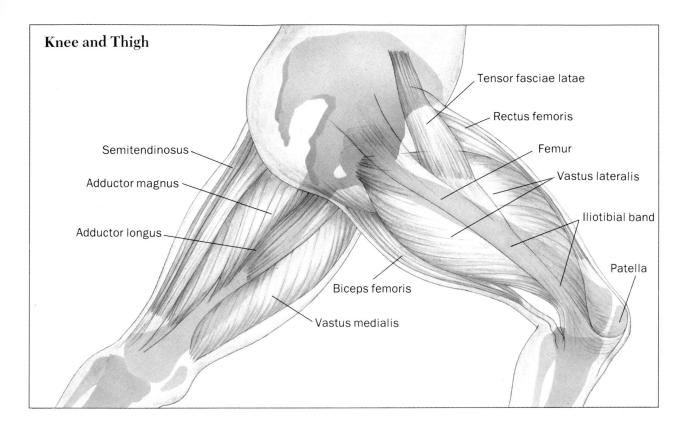

Knee and Thigh

Tensor fasciae latae

Rectus femoris

Femur

Vastus lateralis

Iliotibial band

Patella

Semitendinosus

Adductor magnus

Adductor longus

Biceps femoris

Vastus medialis

from the ages of eight to 15, Osgood-Schlatter disease can be exacerbated by such activities as running and jumping, climbing stairs, weight lifting or doing deep knee bends.

Incorrect form and inadequate conditioning can contribute to knee problems in runners, as can ill-fitting shoes, excessive hill training and increased speeds. Extended aerobic workouts, new dance routines and tennis opponents who make you run round the court more than you are used to can lead to trouble as well. Sometimes the remedies are relatively simple — arch supports for runners, for example, or lower gears and higher seats for cyclists.

Thigh injuries are limited mostly to muscle and tendon strains, particularly in the hamstrings, which tend to shorten and contract, and the adductors, or inner-thigh muscles. Adductor strains, or groin muscle pulls, can be troublesome because many people, even professional athletes, fail to condition the muscles of their inner thighs adequately.

Stress fractures of the thighbone, or femur, which are fairly frequent among the elderly, are rare in younger, healthy individuals. However, many such injuries have been reported among military recruits in basic training and among long-distance runners. Stress fractures of the femur should always be treated by a doctor.

The exercises in this chapter will decrease your chances of sustaining knee and thigh injuries, as well as minimize the everyday aches and pains that occur in this region.

Icing

It is well known that icing reduces pain and speeds recovery time from most stress injuries (*see pages 38-39*). Recent studies also show that icing a joint and reducing its temperature for 30 minute intervals several times a day can produce long-lasting benefits.

Ice packs are more effective than ice massage for lowering the internal temperature of a large joint such as the knee. According to one study, applying an ice pack to a joint for 30 minutes reduced the temperature of the joint for up to four hours. This lowered temperature slows the harmful effects of injury, including swelling, bleeding and the destruction of tissue in a joint.

You can make an ice pack by crushing ice cubes and wrapping them in a damp kitchen towel. Chemical cold packs should be used with caution, since their temperature often drops below freezing, posing a risk of frostbite. If the pack ruptures, the chemicals released may cause skin irritation. It is best to wrap a chemical cold pack in a towel before it is applied to your skin.

Be sure not to leave an ice pack on a joint or other body surface for more than 30 minutes. Also, remove the ice if your skin reddens or if you feel a burning sensation.

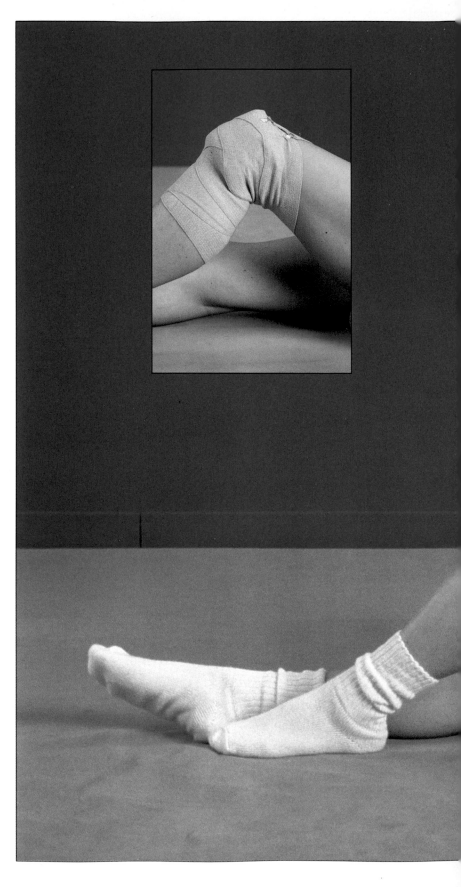

Elevate the injured region above your hip and apply an ice pack wrapped in a towel directly over the injury site *(right)*. **To keep the ice pack from slipping off your knee, apply an elastic bandage** *(inset)*.

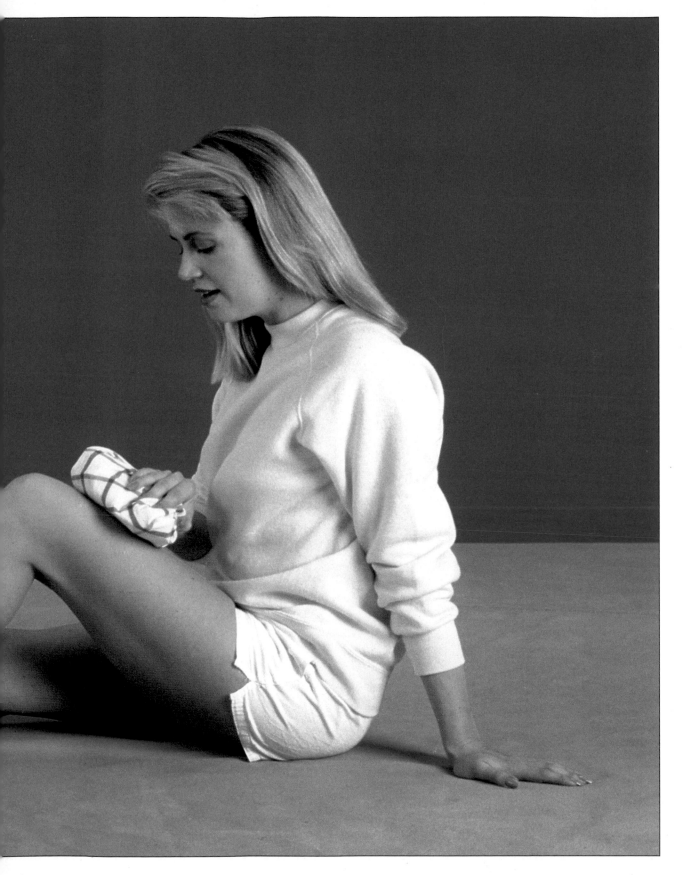

Taping

Although taping supports injured tissues and relieves stress, there is no consensus on which taping technique, if any, is most effective for a particular injury, nor on how long taping can be effective. If it is done incorrectly, the tape may loosen and become practically useless after just a few minutes. If done correctly, however, it should remain effective for at least several hours; depending on the type of taping and its location, it may even provide support for up to a week.

Use adhesive tape against the skin because it provides more support than elastic tape. In addition, elastic tape loosens with use considerably more than adhesive tape does. (Other guidelines for taping are outlined on page 40.) Do not apply adhesive tape directly over cuts or abrasions. Instead, place a dressing over the wound so it will not be aggravated.

If you apply and remove tape often, or if you are applying tape to a particularly sensitive area, position gauze underneath the tape to lessen the chance of skin irritation. You can further reduce the chances of irritation by removing the tape as soon as possible and using rubbing alcohol on the skin to dissolve any remaining adhesive.

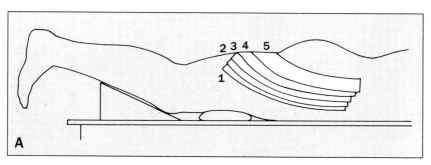

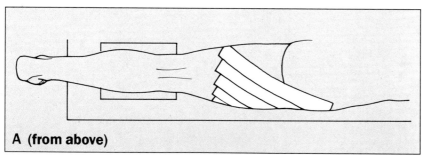

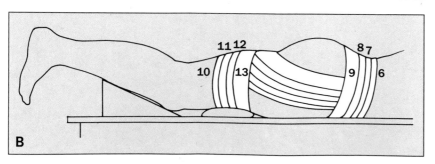

A: To apply tape for a hamstring pull, ask the injured person to lie face down with a small pad under the front of the thigh and with the lower leg supported so that the knee is slightly bent. Apply five overlapping strips of tape, beginning on the outside of the thigh and extending up over the hip. The fifth strip should begin on the inside of the thigh, extend just under the buttocks and end at the hip.
B: Tie down the ends of the strips of tape with four overlapping strips on each end. These tie-down strips should extend almost completely round the limb.

66

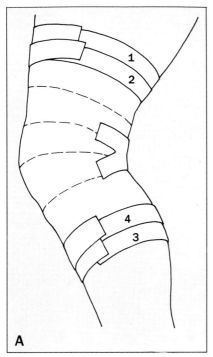

A

To prevent hyperextension of an injured knee, flex it and apply a gauze underwrap. Secure with strips of tape.

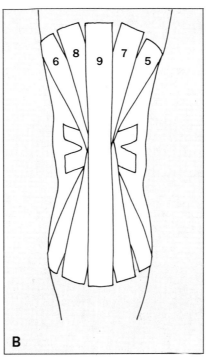

B

Construct a "fan" behind the knee with five strips of tape. Form an X with two strips on the outside first, then fill in.

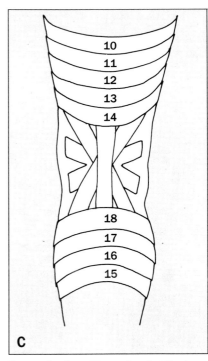

C

Secure the fan with overlapping tie-down strips. Start at the farthest end of the fan first, working your way in.

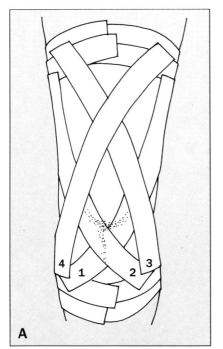

A

To support the knee after a mild sprain, use an underwrap *(top left)*. Apply four overlapping strips from the lower leg to the thigh, leaving the kneecap exposed.

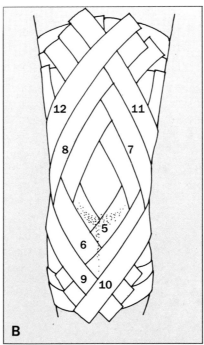

B

Continue the procedure with six more strips of tape, beginning on the lower leg and crossing over to the thigh. Again, the kneecap should be exposed in the centre.

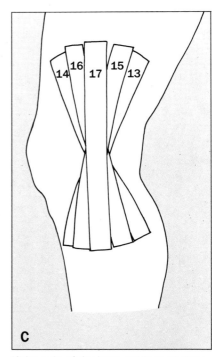

C

If the pain of the knee strain is on one side of the knee, apply a fan on that side. Make an X with two strips of tape and fill in the form. Secure with tie-down strips.

67

Hamstrings/1

Composed of three distinct muscles, the hamstrings run from the back of the hip-bone to the back of the knee, where they connect with the tibia and the fibula, the bones of the lower leg. The hamstrings enable you to extend your hips and flex your knees.

Hamstring injuries can be among the most debilitating of athletic injuries. Once these muscles have been pulled or torn, they tend to present recurring problems. This is partly because the hamstrings are opposed by the more powerful quadriceps on the front of the thigh; this imbalance tends to strain the hamstrings and predispose them to further injury.

Hamstring tendinitis, or soreness in the hamstring tendons behind the knee, may result from tight or weak hamstrings or from running down-hill. Tight hamstrings can also cause pain in the back, since the shortened muscles will keep the pelvis tilted backwards, stressing the lower spine.

You can condition your hamstrings by running with short, quick strides. Alternate with more vigorous sprinting and kicking your heels up as high as possible. Another conditioning technique is to cycle in low gear but with a high cadence, or pedalling rate. In order to strengthen or rehabilitate your hamstrings, do the exercises on these two pages. Perform three sets of 10 repetitions of exercises done with either the ankle weights or the elastic exercise band. Be sure to exercise each leg. Then stretch your hamstrings with the exercises on pages 70-71.

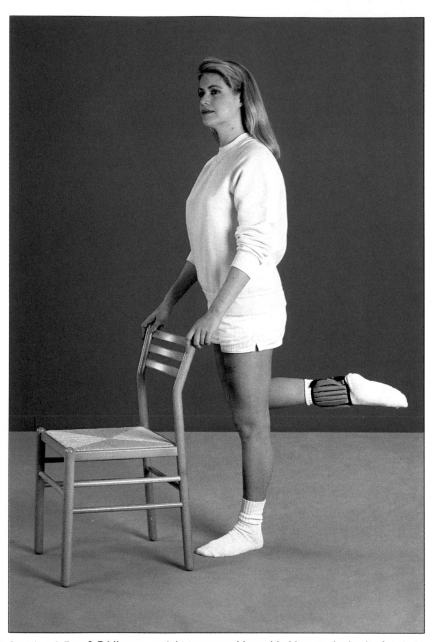

Attach a 1.5 to 2.5 kilogram weight to your ankle and hold on to the back of a chair or some other stationary object. Lift your heel towards your buttocks, then lower your foot to the floor. Repeat with your other foot.

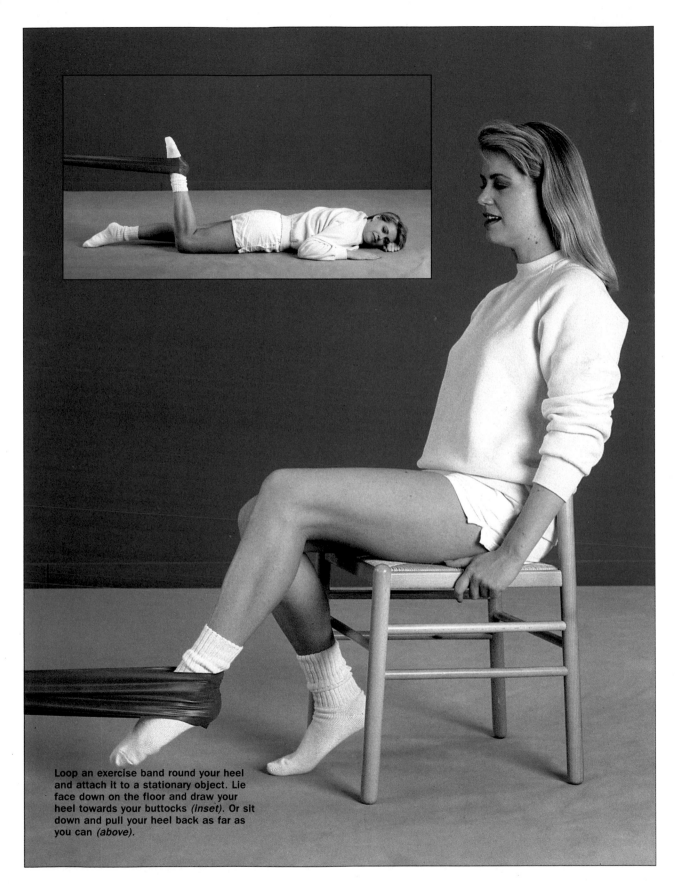

Loop an exercise band round your heel and attach it to a stationary object. Lie face down on the floor and draw your heel towards your buttocks *(inset)*. Or sit down and pull your heel back as far as you can *(above)*.

Hamstrings/2

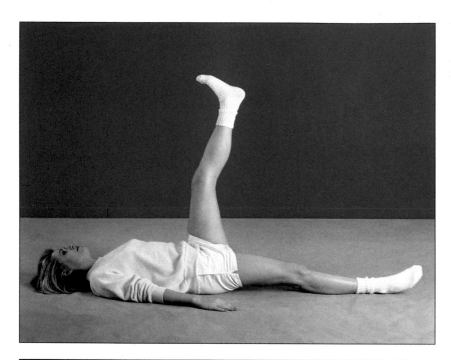

To stretch your hamstrings, lie on your back with your legs extended. Lift one leg towards the ceiling *(left)*, and then try to straighten your leg. Hold for at least 20 seconds. Repeat with the other leg.

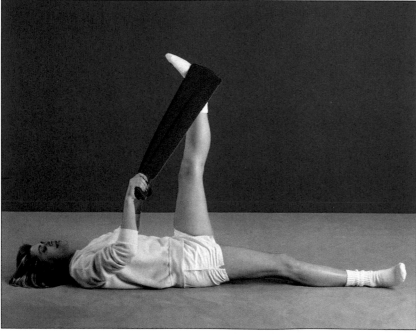

For a more powerful stretch, lie on your back with your legs extended and loop a towel round your left heel. Keeping your knee straight, lift your foot towards the ceiling, pulling on the towel to produce the stretch *(left)*. Hold for at least 20 seconds and repeat with your right leg.

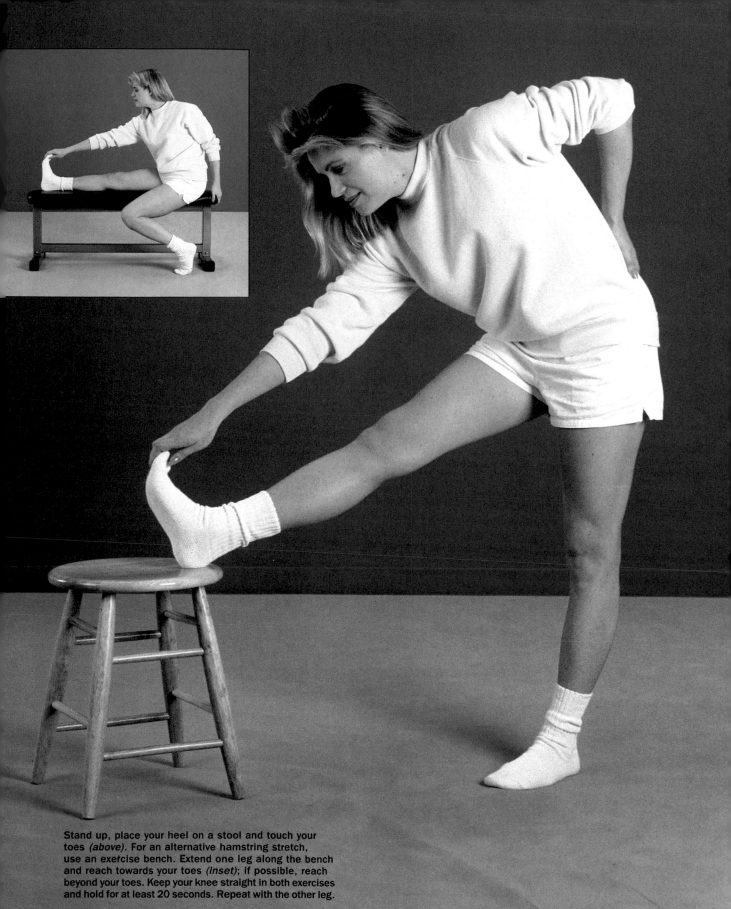

Stand up, place your heel on a stool and touch your toes *(above)*. For an alternative hamstring stretch, use an exercise bench. Extend one leg along the bench and reach towards your toes *(inset)*; if possible, reach beyond your toes. Keep your knee straight in both exercises and hold for at least 20 seconds. Repeat with the other leg.

71

Quadriceps/1

The quadriceps is a group of four muscles that extend down the front of your thigh, joining in a single tendon that inserts into your kneecap. One muscle in the group, the rectus femoris, originates in your pelvis; the others originate from various points along the thighbone. These muscles, usually the most powerful in your body, are absolutely crucial to any activity that involves walking, running, jumping or just standing.

You can test the strength of your rectus femoris by standing on one leg and lifting your other leg up with your knee straight. Hold that leg as high as you can. The longer you can hold your leg up, the stronger your rectus femoris. You will feel a burning sensation along your thigh when this muscle becomes fatigued.

Together, all of the four quadriceps muscles act to straighten the knee and guide the kneecap in its groove at the end of the thighbone. Weak or inflexible quadriceps may lead to incorrect tracking of the kneecap and contribute to patellofemoral pain, or runner's knee, one of the most common knee injuries.

The exercises on these two pages will strengthen your quadriceps. If you do not have an exercise band, you can substitute the exercises on pages 74-75. Perform three sets of 10 repetitions of a quadriceps exercise for each leg. Turn to page 77 for stretching exercises.

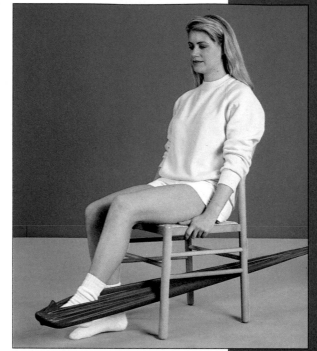

Attach an exercise band to a stationary object. Sit on a chair and loop the band round one foot *(above)*. Raise your lower leg until your knee is straight, then return to the starting position.

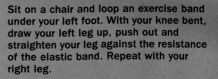

Sit on a chair and loop an exercise band under your left foot. With your knee bent, draw your left leg up, push out and straighten your leg against the resistance of the elastic band. Repeat with your right leg.

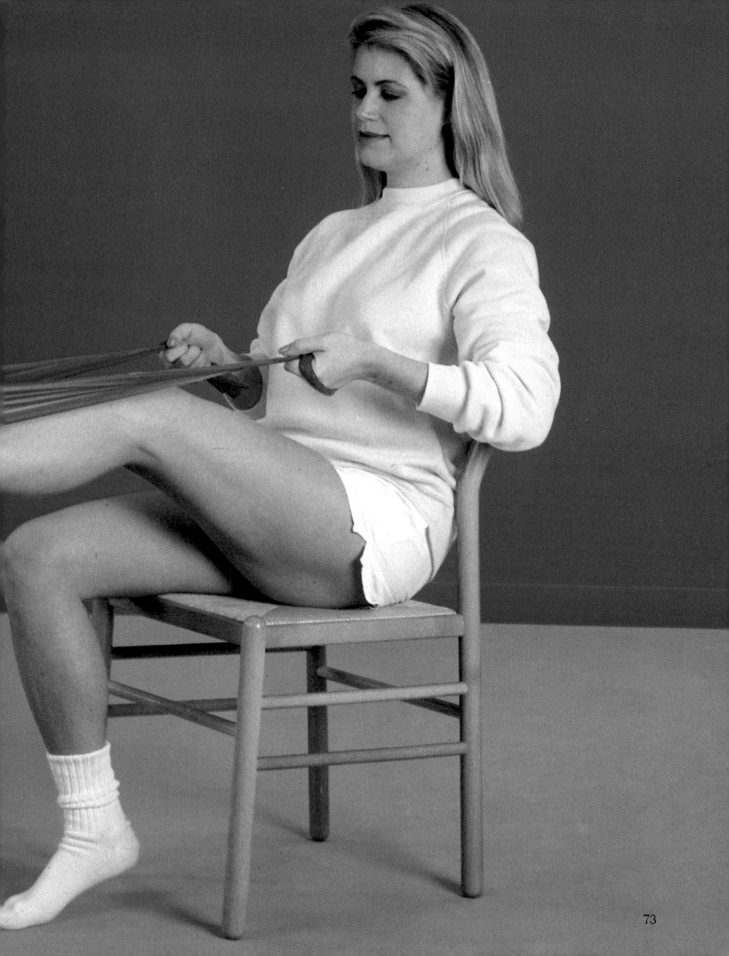

Quadriceps/2

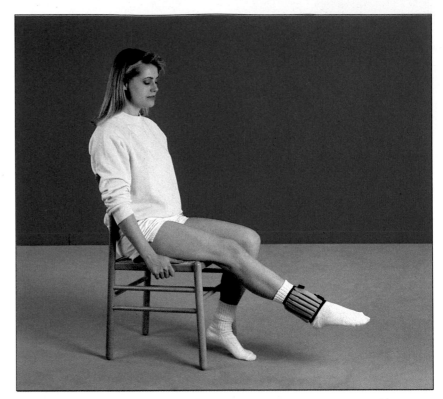

Attach an ankle weight to your right leg and sit on a chair with both feet on the floor. Raise your right leg until it is straight. Repeat with your left leg.

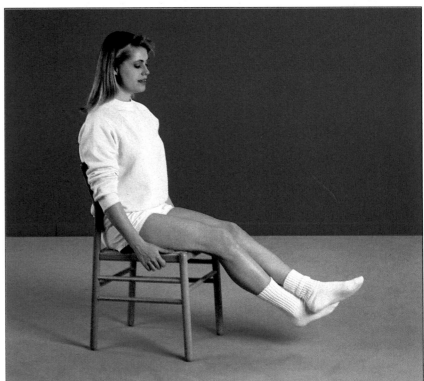

If you do not have an ankle weight for the above exercise, place your left foot over your right ankle. Straighten your right knee, lifting your left leg. Switch feet and repeat for your left leg.

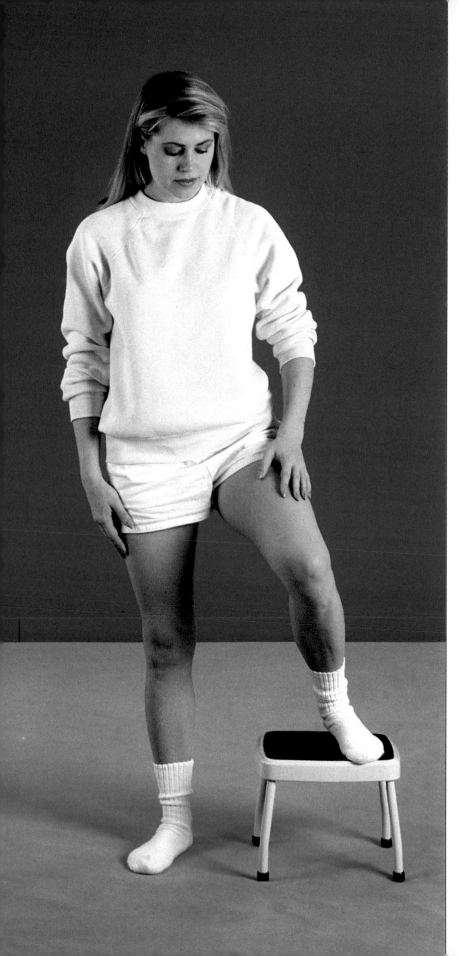

Stand next to a low stool and step up and down with your left leg. Turn round and repeat with your right leg.

Quadriceps/3

Assume a sitting position against a wall with your upper and lower legs forming a right angle. Stay in this position for as long as you can. Time yourself. The stronger your quadriceps become, the longer you will be able to maintain the position.

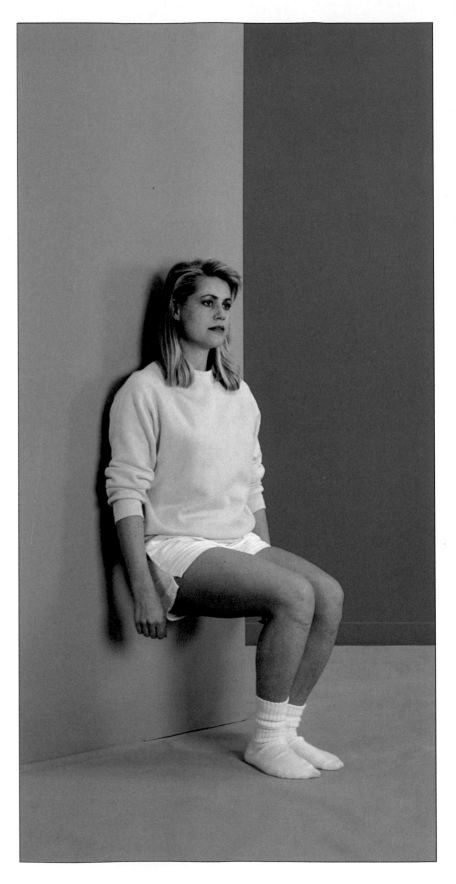

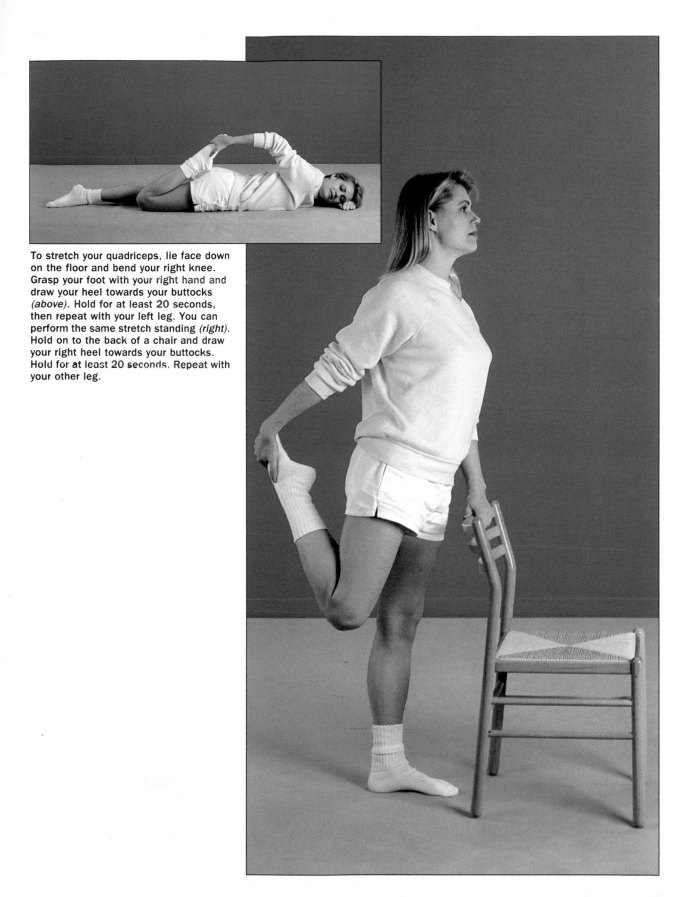

To stretch your quadriceps, lie face down on the floor and bend your right knee. Grasp your foot with your right hand and draw your heel towards your buttocks *(above)*. Hold for at least 20 seconds, then repeat with your left leg. You can perform the same stretch standing *(right)*. Hold on to the back of a chair and draw your right heel towards your buttocks. Hold for at least 20 seconds. Repeat with your other leg.

Hip Flexors/1

The hip flexors are a group of muscles that bend the hip and lift the thigh. If you move your knee towards your torso you are lifting your thigh with your hip flexors. When your legs are fixed, you use your hip flexors to help you perform sit-ups.

Although the hip flexors all originate in the hip, they are a diverse group. Some attach to the lower spine; others attach to the thighbone. One of the hip-flexor muscles is the rectus femoris, which attaches to the kneecap and which is also included in the quadriceps group. The flexor known as the sartorius is the longest muscle in the body. It extends in an S curve from the outside of the hipbone, along the inside of the thigh, across the inside of the knee joint, where it attaches to the shinbone below the kneecap. Among its many functions, the sartorius allows you to cross your legs.

Weak or tight hip-flexor muscles can result in knee problems and pain in the lower back. Inflexible hip flexors can cause the pelvis to rotate or tilt forwards, causing lordosis, or excessive curvature of the spine. This condition also leads to posture resembling that of a person with a pot belly. You can correct these problems with stretching exercises for the hip flexor muscles *(pages 82-83)* and strengthening exercises for the abdominal muscles *(page 118)*.

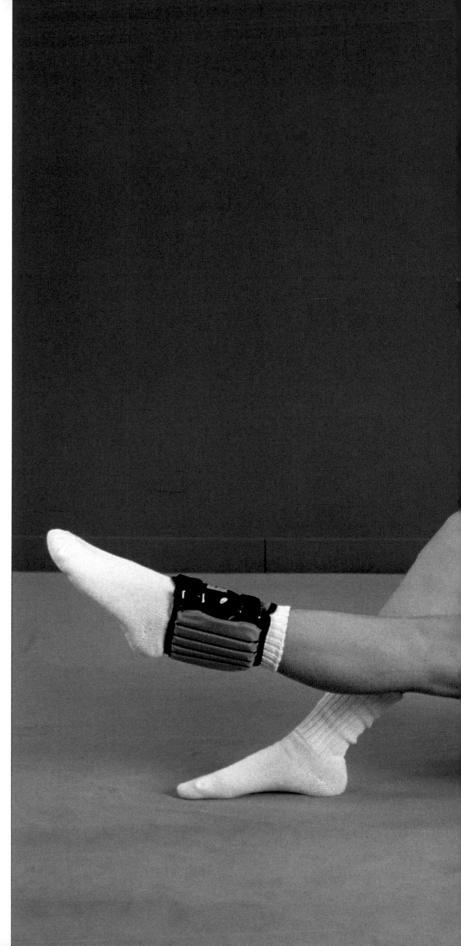

Lie on your back with one leg extended. Keeping your knee straight, lift the extended leg for three sets of 10 repetitions *(inset)*. When your hip flexors become stronger, perform the same exercise using ankle weights *(right)*.

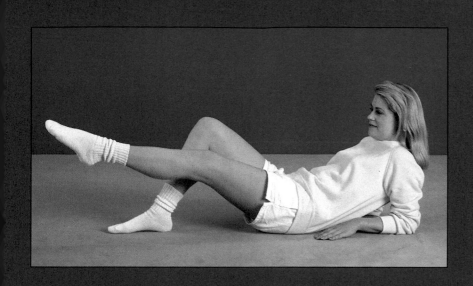

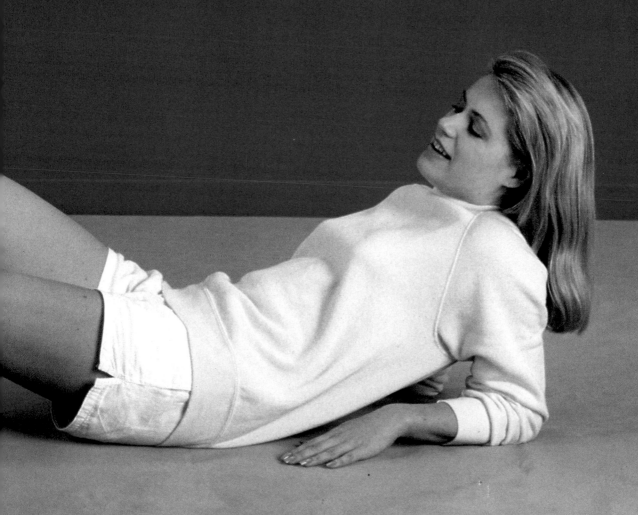

Hip Flexors/2

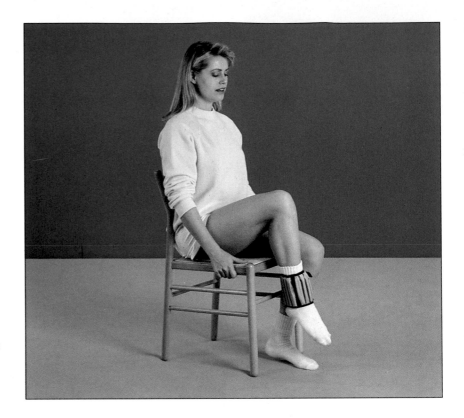

Sit on a chair and attach an ankle weight to one leg. Hold on to the chair to keep your hips in place and raise your knee for three sets of 10 repetitions. Repeat with the other leg.

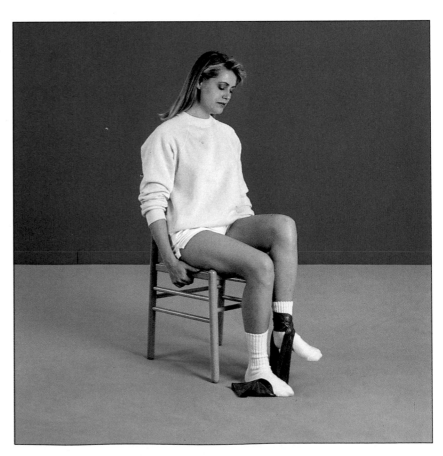

For a variation of the above exercise, wrap an elastic exercise band round your left ankle and step on the end of the band with your right foot. Raise your left knee. Perform three sets of 10 repetitions. Repeat with your other leg.

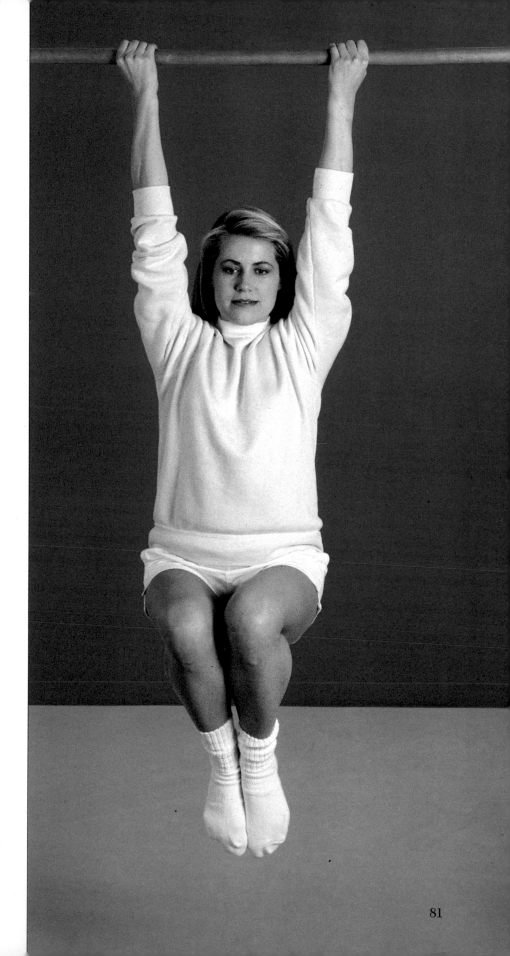

Hang on a chinning bar and draw your knees up so that your thighs are parallel to the floor. You can test the strength of your hip flexors by seeing how long you can hold this position.

81

Hip Flexors/3

To stretch your hip flexors, stand with your back to an exercise bench or low stool. Bend one knee back and place the top of your foot on the bench. Then bend your other knee until you feel a stretch. Hold for at least 20 seconds and repeat with your other leg.

Lie face down on the floor and bend one knee, grasping your foot and drawing your heel towards your buttocks. Be sure that your knee and thigh are slightly elevated. Hold for 20 seconds and repeat with the other leg.

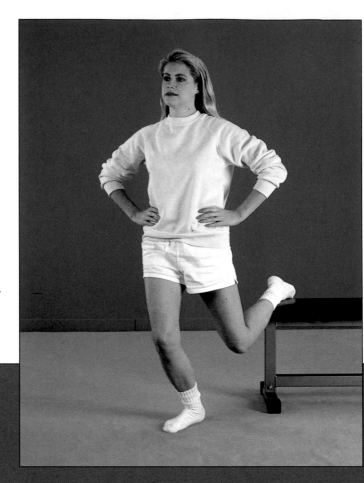

Lie face up on an exercise bench with your right knee drawn towards your chest. Grasp the knee with your right hand. Extend your left leg over the end of the bench and pull on your foot with your left hand, stretching the left hip flexors for at least 20 seconds. Switch leg positions and repeat.

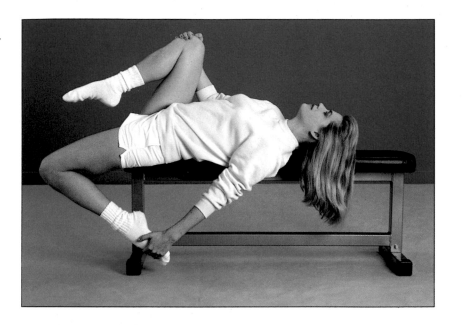

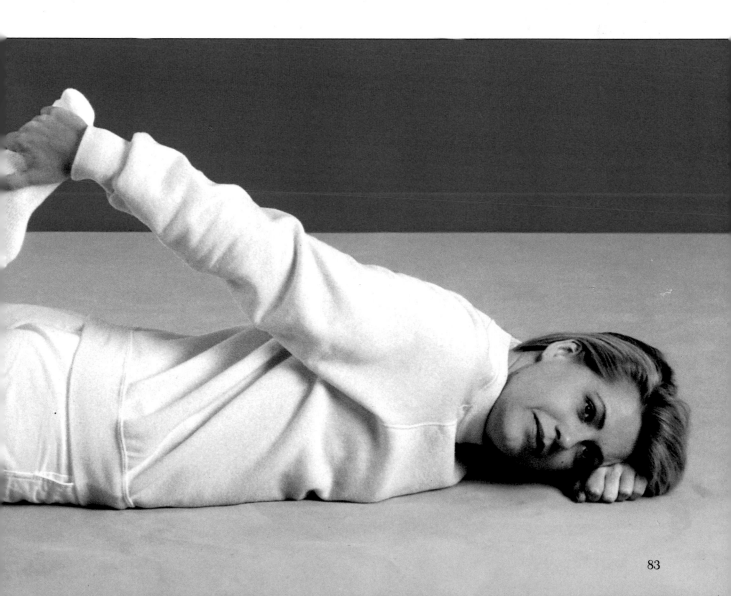

Gluteals

Opposing the hip flexors, which draw the thigh forwards, are the hip extensors, which pull the thigh backwards. The hip extensors include the hamstrings (*see pages 68-71*) and the gluteals, or buttocks muscles. While the hamstrings extend the hip and flex the knee, the gluteals apply their force more directly to the thigh. The largest buttocks muscle, called the gluteus maximus, is one of the most powerful muscles in the body.

For all its strength, though, the gluteus maximus is not used as often as the hamstrings or the quadriceps.

Electromyographic studies, which are tracings of the electrical stimulation of muscles, indicate that the gluteus maximus is not essential for walking on level ground, but that it does, however, perform an important function when you are walking up an incline or gradient. By bending forwards from the hip at the beginning of a race, a sprinter uses the gluteus maximus for a great burst of energy off the starting block.

Studies on the effects of contracting the gluteus maximus have produced surprising results. When you stand erect with your feet parallel and pinch your buttocks together, for instance, your gluteus maximus causes a slight external rotation of the hip joint, turns your legs slightly, and causes your feet to rotate outwards and the inside of your arch to lift. Contracting the muscles in your buttocks also lessens curvature in your lower back, and in addition, strengthening the gluteals will improve your posture.

You can strengthen your hip extensors by running up hills or jumping up and down on one leg. You can also perform the exercises on these two pages.

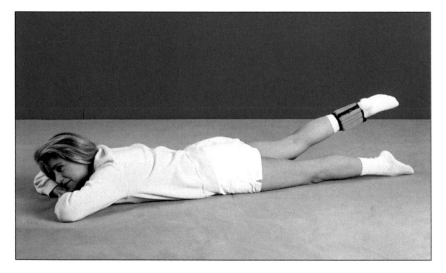

Lie face down on the floor and attach ankle weights to one leg. Keeping your knee straight, lift your leg for three sets of 10 repetitions. Switch legs. Repeat.

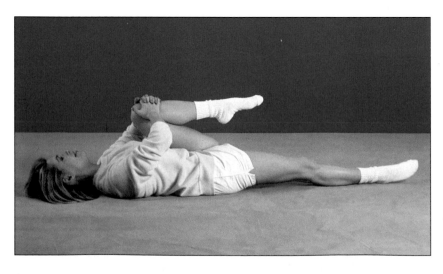

To stretch the hip extensors, lie on your back and bend one knee. Grasp the knee and draw it towards your chest. Hold for at least 20 seconds, then repeat with the other leg.

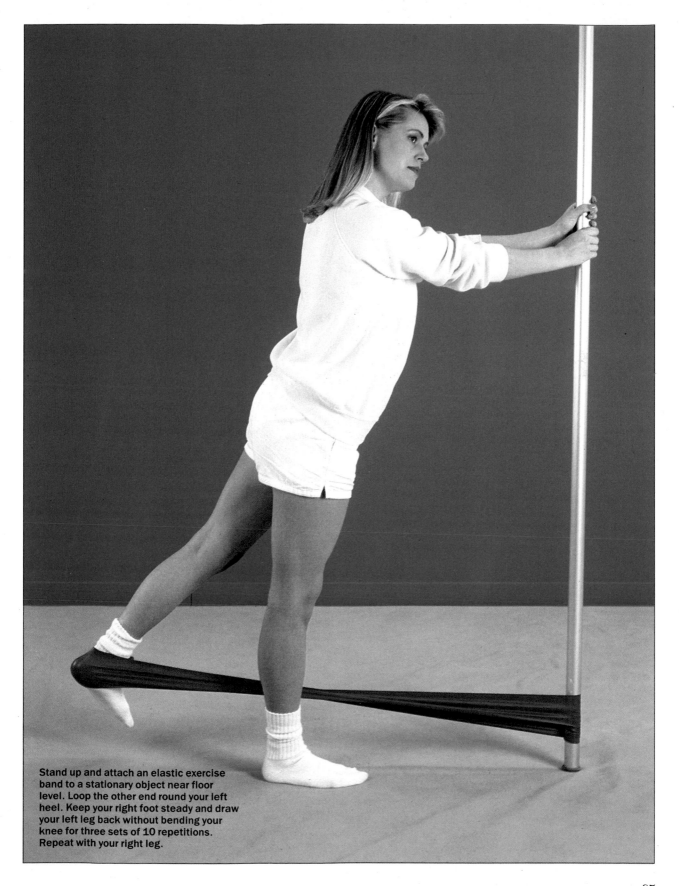

Stand up and attach an elastic exercise band to a stationary object near floor level. Loop the other end round your left heel. Keep your right foot steady and draw your left leg back without bending your knee for three sets of 10 repetitions. Repeat with your right leg.

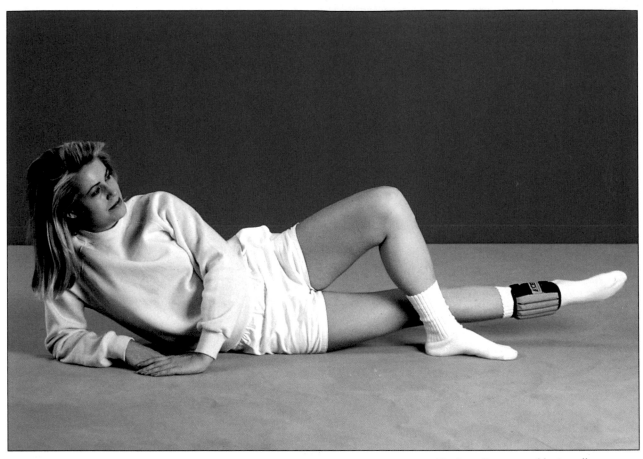

To strengthen your adductors, lie on your right side and attach an ankle weight to your right leg. Cross your left leg over your right and place your left foot flat on the floor as shown above. Keeping your right leg extended, lift it off the floor. Perform three sets of 10 leg lifts. Turn over and repeat for the left leg.

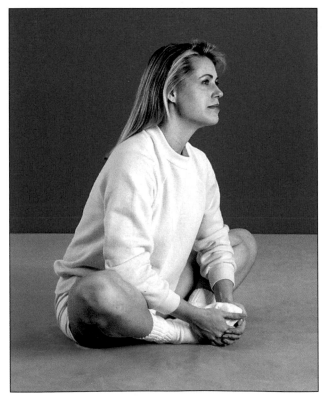

To stretch the adductors, sit cross-legged on the floor, then bring the soles of your feet together. Grasp your feet with your hands and lean forwards with your back straight. Hold for at least 20 seconds.

Adductors

The adductors, or muscles of the groin, originate from the pubic bone and attach along a strip running down the thighbone. These muscles act to pull your legs in towards each other. The adductors enable a rider to straddle and remain mounted on a horse. When you run, the adductors work to help pull your rear leg forwards after it leaves the ground.

Overexertion of the adductors and groin-muscle pulls most often occur during sprinting, especially since most people — even athletes — fail to condition their adductor muscles adequately. Since the adductors also help keep your toes from pointing outwards, running on a surface that is slippery, such as wet grass or snow-covered streets, can result in groin-muscle strain. Groin-muscle pulls can be painful and tend to recur; the best precaution against such injury is to perform strengthening and stretching exercises for the adductors, as shown on these pages.

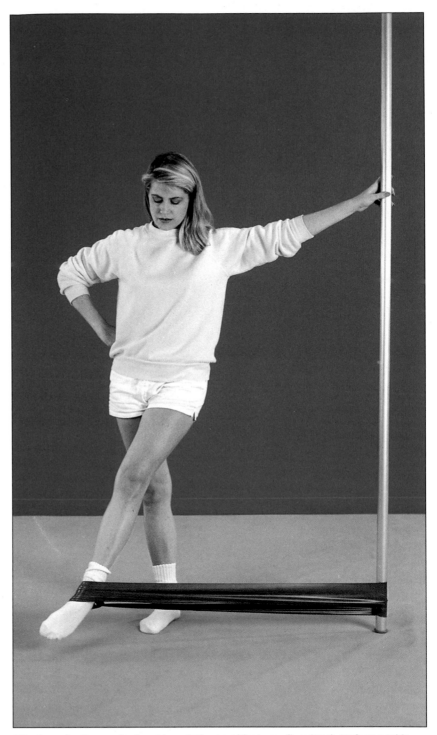

Attach an elastic exercise band to a stationary object near floor level, such as a table leg. Stand with the band to your left and loop the end round your left ankle. Hold on to something for stability, swing your left leg inwards and across your right for three sets of 10 repetitions. Turn round and repeat for your right leg.

Abductors

The abductors oppose the adductors and work to swing the leg outwards, away from the medial line of the body. The chief abductors are the gluteus medius, or intermediate buttocks muscle, and the gluteus minimus, or small buttocks muscle. In addition to abducting the thigh — drawing it away from the body — these muscles hold your hip in place when you walk, stabilizing your upper body and allowing you to transfer your weight smoothly from foot to foot.

The outward rotation of the thigh is also affected by several small muscles that attach to the hip from the top of the femur. The sciatic nerve runs over, or sometimes even through, one of these muscles, the piriformis. If the piriformis becomes irritated or too tight, it can pinch the sciatic nerve. Because this nerve is the largest one in the body, supplying sensation to much of the leg from the hip down, a pinched sciatic nerve can cause pain, numbness or a tingling sensation from the buttocks to the foot. This uncomfortable condition is commonly called sciatica. You can relieve or prevent sciatica that is associated with exercise, and condition your abductors, with the stretching exercise on this page.

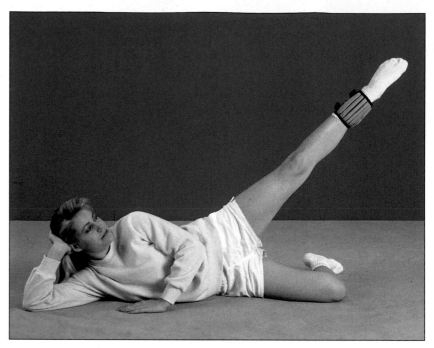

To strengthen your abductors, lie on your right side and attach an ankle weight to your left leg. Bend your right knee for stability and keep your hips perpendicular to the floor. With your left leg extended, raise your foot towards the ceiling for three sets of 10 repetitions. Turn over and repeat for your right leg.

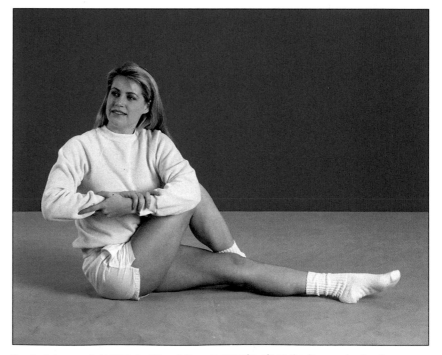

To stretch your abductors and the piriformis muscle, sit on the floor and extend your left leg. Cross your right leg over it and draw your right knee back with your left arm. Hold for at least 20 seconds and repeat for your other leg.

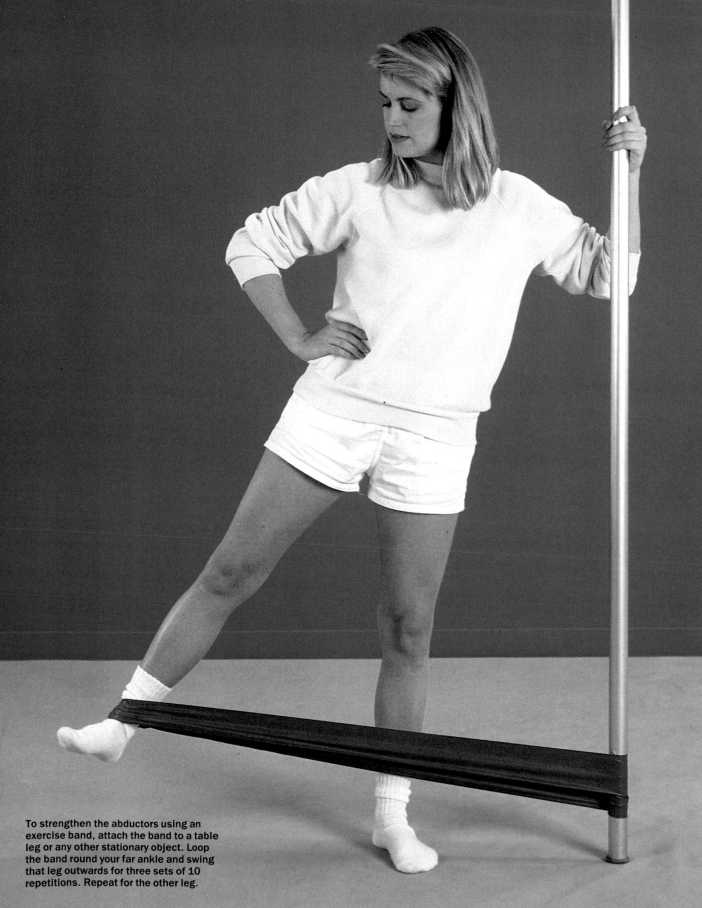

To strengthen the abductors using an exercise band, attach the band to a table leg or any other stationary object. Loop the band round your far ankle and swing that leg outwards for three sets of 10 repetitions. Repeat for the other leg.

Iliotibial Band

The iliotibial band is a tendon that acts like a tense ligament, running down the outside of the thigh and attaching just below the outside of the knee. It helps to stabilize the knee joint.

People who often run downhill, who pronate excessively or who run on one side of the road so that the kerb-side leg is stressed more than the other can develop iliotibial-band-friction syndrome. Inflammation and swelling occur when the band becomes irritated from rubbing across the bone on the outside of the knee. People who are bow-legged, who have leg-length discrepancies or who have high arches are also prone to iliotibial band problems. You can also get this injury from walking up stairs a lot. It begins as a slight discomfort on the outside of the knee and can progress to an excruciating burning sensation.

Iliotibial-band-friction syndrome is difficult to eliminate once it has reached an advanced stage. If you begin to feel discomfort just below the outside of your knee, therefore, you should be careful not to irritate the region further. Rest and ice massage are very effective remedies. The stretching exercises shown here will help prevent iliotibial problems.

Lie on your back with your left leg extended. Cross your right leg over your left and place your foot flat on the floor. Grasp your knee with your left hand and draw it towards the floor. Hold for at least 20 seconds and repeat with the left leg.

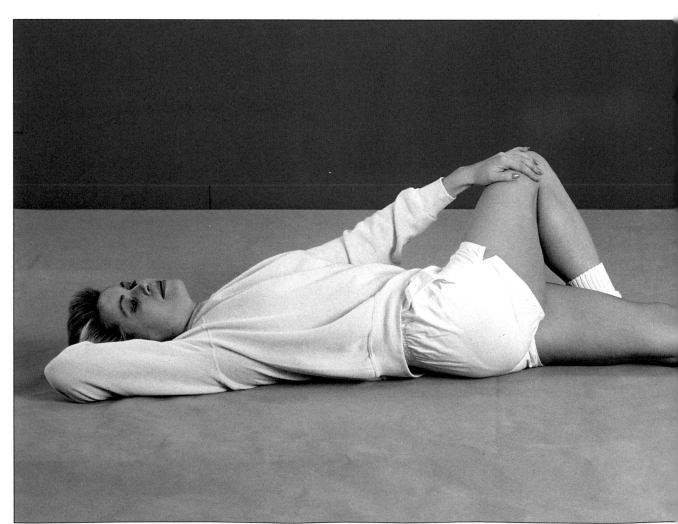

Cross your right leg over your left and place your right foot on the floor. Being careful to maintain your balance, lean to the left to stretch the right iliotibial band. Hold for at least 20 seconds, then repeat on the other side.

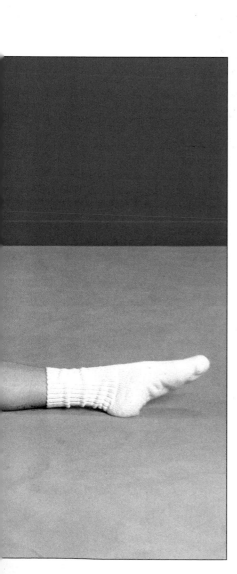

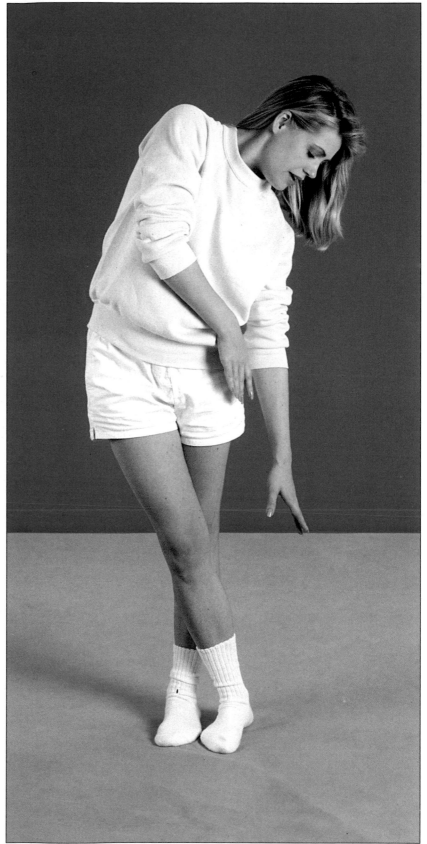

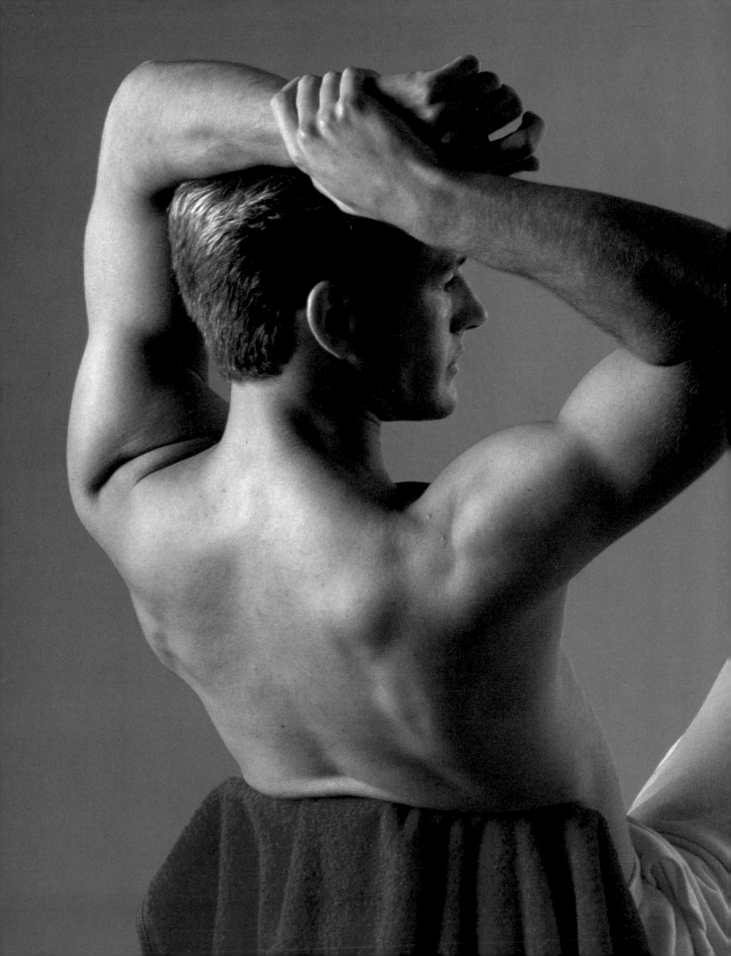

CHAPTER FOUR

The Upper Body

*Coping with the varied demands
on your back, shoulders,
elbows and wrists*

Rest and rehabilitation are the keys to recovery for many upper body injuries, especially for injuries to the shoulder, the body's strongest and most flexible, but least stable, joint. For years, however, coaches and doctors tended to underestimate the importance of exercise for recuperation from these injuries. If rest did not produce the desired recovery in such athletes as cricket fast bowlers, who are prone to shoulder strains from throwing too many fast balls, the next step would often be to operate on the injured muscles. But sports-medicine experts have recently become aware that rest must be accompanied by a gradual build-up of exercise to stretch and strengthen the injured muscles; otherwise the muscles may atrophy from disuse, making their recovery much more difficult.

The shoulder's ball-shaped head rotates in a shallow cup in the shoulder blade. Unlike the knee, another frequently injured joint, the shoulder is not secured by strong ligaments. The ligaments that keep the shoulder in place can only withstand a force of about 45 to 75 kilograms, but the impact from a fall or collision can easily load the shoulders with much more force than this. When the force placed on a shoulder exceeds the strength of its ligaments, the surrounding ligaments can avoid being injured only by absorbing the excess. Fortunately, the shoulder is stabilized by four tendons that comprise the rotator cuff and by a number of powerful muscles, including the biceps, the triceps, the deltoid, the latissimus dorsi and the pectoralis major. But even this array of musculature cannot totally protect the shoulder from stress injuries. Swimming, throwing and golfing, all of which make different demands on the upper body, can cause similar problems for the shoulder joint. Whenever your shoulder repeatedly makes wide, sweeping arcs while your arm is exerting propulsive force, there is some risk of injury.

Supporting not just your shoulders but your entire upper body is a single anatomical unit — the spinal column. Though the 24 movable vertebrae of the spine support the entire upper body, the back does not remain rigid but instead must bend and twist in many directions. For this reason, it is curvilinear in design, forming an S as it extends from the neck down through the rib cage, where it is called the thoracic spine, to the lower back, or lumbar spine. The cervical area — your neck — has the greatest mobility. It is also the part of the spinal column most vulnerable to acute injury. One such injury is whiplash, a sprain of the cervical spine resulting from a sudden sharp whipping movement of the head and neck, which may happen in a car accident. Cervical sprains are extremely painful because the neck muscles go into spasm to prevent movement and protect the ligaments from further injury. Medical treatment may include muscle relaxants and painkillers for the spasm, as well as a collar for the sprain.

Despite its having the largest vertebrae and the most powerful supporting muscles, the lower back is where many back problems arise. Baseball, basketball and rugby players are all vulnerable to lumbar muscle strain from any quick twists and turns, as are dancers. And almost everyone is subject to lower back pain at some time.

Your spinal column is supported by the spine muscles and opposing abdominals, and the two muscle groups should be balanced in strength. The spine muscles are naturally strong in most people, but the abdominals, if not toned and strengthened systematically, are weak; therefore, one of the best ways to guard against or alleviate back problems is to strengthen your abdominal muscles with exercise.

Strengthening exercise is also the best way to cope with other upper body problems, such as tennis elbow, a type of tendinitis that is one of the most common stress injuries of the arm. Studies have shown that tennis elbow affects almost one third of all players; regular players over the age of 40 are the most likely to be bothered. There are two types of tennis elbow. The lateral version, which affects the outside of the joint, is often the result of performing backhand strokes

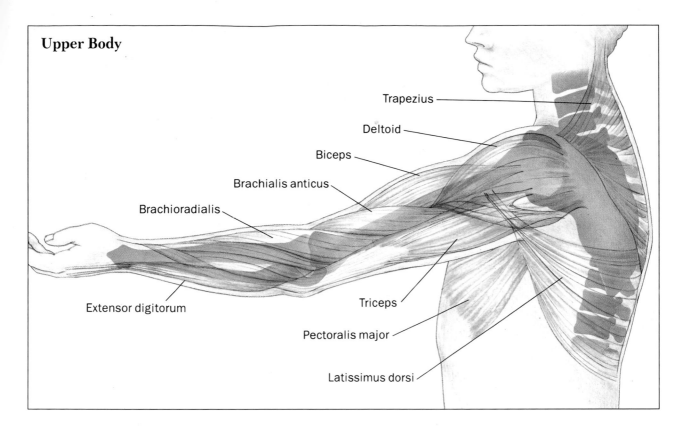

Upper Body

Trapezius

Deltoid

Biceps

Brachialis anticus

Brachioradialis

Extensor digitorum

Triceps

Pectoralis major

Latissimus dorsi

incorrectly. For instance, if you snap your wrist to give more drive to the ball, you place stress on the forearm muscles that attach to a bony knob on the outside of your elbow, producing tendinitis at that point. By using a racket that is too heavy or that has too large a grip for your hand, you further stress these muscles. Performing forehand strokes incorrectly can affect the inner forearm, resulting in a condition known as medial tennis elbow. Exercising to strengthen the supporting arm muscles effectively treats and prevents both types of injury.

The wrist and hand are subject to injuries ranging from minor cuts to serious sprains and fractures. The wrist consists of a packet of eight small bones wrapped in ligaments. Underneath are the two main forearm bones, the ulna and the radius. Although the wrist has the ability to bend easily, its main function is providing stability for the hand, whose power comes primarily from the muscles in the forearm. All sports activities that involve repeated forceful arm movements — tennis, volleyball, ten pin bowling and weight training, among others — can lead to tendinitis in the wrist. Even gardening has been known to produce this type of injury.

This chapter includes exercises designed to strengthen and protect all the important tendons, ligaments, bones and joints in the upper body. Such exercises can also help speed recovery when injuries, aches or pains do occur; however, any injury that causes intense pain, or long-lasting aches, or other symptoms that concern you, should be diagnosed and treated by a doctor.

Taping/1

Adhesive taping can be an effective way to stabilize a joint and protect an injury from stress so that it has a chance to recover quickly. Taping the hand joints, the wrist and the elbow can be particularly effective because these regions have little fat and connective tissue. Fat and connective tissue allow the skin to slide backwards and forwards over the underlying tissue, which significantly reduces the effectiveness of the taping.

Wash your skin and shave body hair from the area to be taped. Apply a protective gauze underwrapping if you need to tape an area of the body that you do not wish to shave or if you are allergic to adhesive tape.

Be careful when removing tape. Use only bandage scissors or specially designed tape cutters to avoid injury. Do not rip the tape off, but slowly peel it from your skin. Once you have removed the tape, wash the skin with soap and water to clean off the adhesive residue. If the skin is dry, apply a moisturizer.

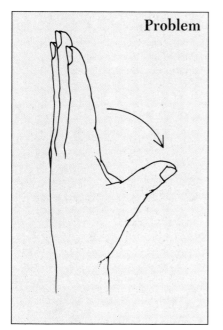

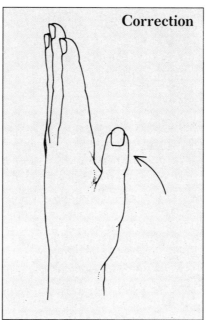

Abduction injuries to the thumb *(far left)* occur when the thumb is pulled back forcefully from the palm and fingers. This commonly happens to skiers holding poles when they fall and to ice hockey players whose sticks get trapped. To prepare the thumb for taping, place it in a neutral position *(left)*.

A: Apply tape in a figure-of-eight pattern by starting on the back of the wrist; loop under the wrist, round the thumb and up over the back of the wrist again to start the second figure-of-eight. Overlap four figures-of-eight. *B:* Anchor the figures-of-eight with two overlapping tie-downs on the wrist.

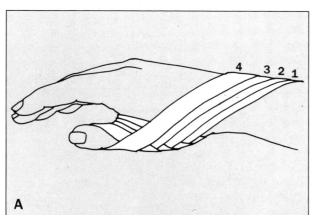

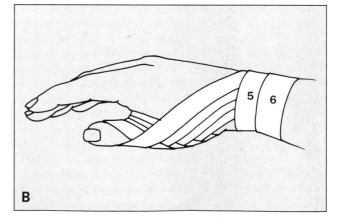

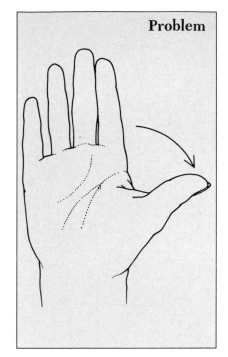

Problem

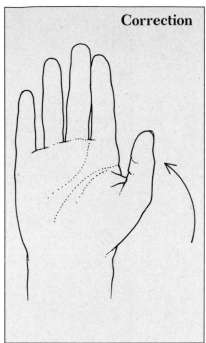

Correction

Extension injuries to the thumb *(far left)* occur when the thumb is pulled too far to the side, away from the fingers. This can happen in a collision with another player in a team sport. Move the thumb to a neutral position *(left)* to prepare for taping.

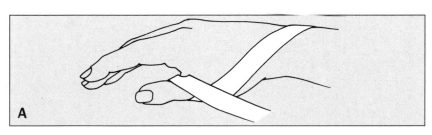

A

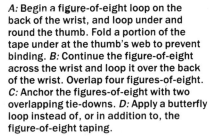

A: Begin a figure-of-eight loop on the back of the wrist, and loop under and round the thumb. Fold a portion of the tape under at the thumb's web to prevent binding. *B:* Continue the figure-of-eight across the wrist and loop it over the back of the wrist. Overlap four figures-of-eight. *C:* Anchor the figures-of-eight with two overlapping tie-downs. *D:* Apply a butterfly loop instead of, or in addition to, the figure-of-eight taping.

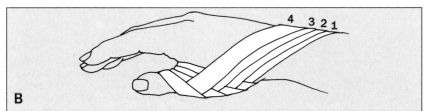

4 3 2 1

B

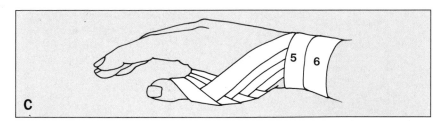

5 6

C

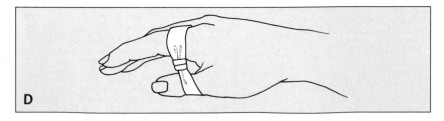

D

97

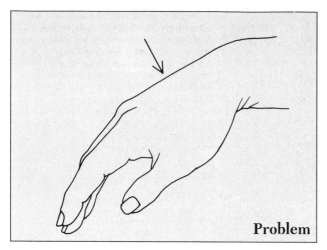

Problem

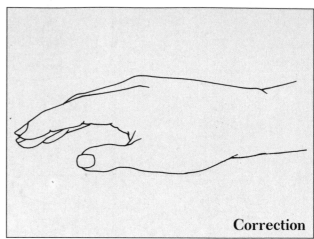

Correction

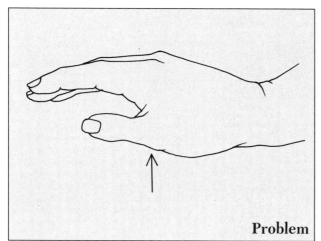

Problem

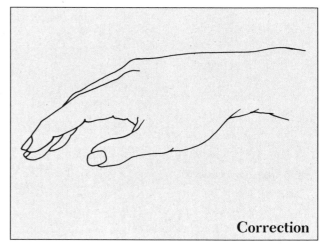

Correction

Taping/2

A hyperflexion injury to the wrist *(top left)* occurs when your palm is forced towards your forearm, resulting in a mild sprain. Correct it for taping by moving your hand back in a slightly extended position *(top right)*. A hyperextension wrist injury *(above left)* is a common occurrence after a fall. Keep the wrist in a slightly flexed position *(above)* to prepare it for taping.

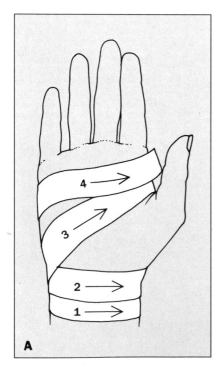

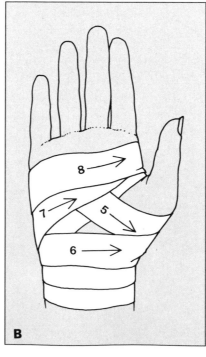

A: To support the wrist and limit its range of motion following a mild sprain, begin taping at the top of the wrist and loop twice round the wrist. Wrap the third and fourth loops across the palm, being sure not to make the tape too tight. *B:* Continue four more loops of the tape round the palm, wrist and thumb.

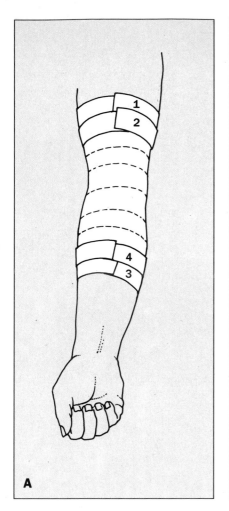

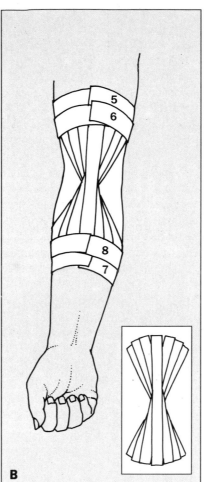

A: For a hyperextension injury in which the elbow is bent back as in a fall or collision, resulting in a mild sprain, keep the elbow slightly flexed and apply an underwrap of gauze, securing the ends with adhesive tape. *B:* Construct a fan out of seven 20-centimetre strips of tape *(inset)*. Apply the fan over the gauze and tie down both ends with two strips of adhesive tape to secure the fan. Once the tape is applied, you should be able to bend your elbow but not extend it fully.

Hand

Because you use them instinctively to break falls and avoid or cushion collisions, your hands may be subject to any number of injuries. And because the joints in your hands are so small, even minor swelling there can cause a great deal of discomfort. A jammed finger, for instance, can be painful for weeks. Dislocations of the finger and thumb require medical attention.

Although the structure of the hand is very much like that of the foot, the hand is far more flexible than the foot, mainly because it does not have to bear any weight. The four fingers have considerable flexion and extension, the ability to curl and point; the thumb can also move in and out and rotate in circles.

Skier's thumb — stretched or torn ligaments at the thumb's base — is the most common thumb injury. It often occurs as a result of falling on your hand when your thumb is outstretched, or your thumb getting twisted back by the ski pole while downhill skiing. Treat mild cases of skier's thumb as you would any other sprain — with rest, ice and compression *(page 24)*. Then, when the pain and swelling subside, begin a gentle stretching and exercise programme. Severe skier's thumb can be a debilitating injury, so if you have any doubt about your condition, you should consult a doctor.

Many of the muscles that control hand and finger movements are actually in the forearm, not in the hand, and are connected to the fingers by long tendons. You can improve the strength and the flexibility of these muscles, and so lessen your chances of injury, by performing the exercises on this and the opposite page.

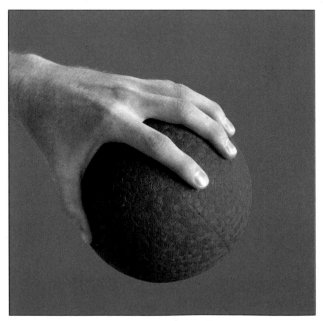

Grip a large rubber ball as hard as you can for a second, then relax. Perform three sets of 10 repetitions, then switch hands.

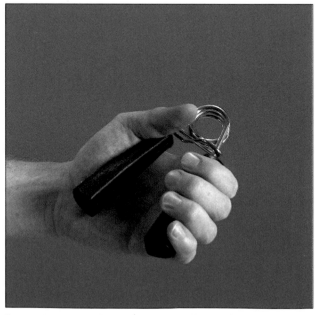

For a variation, grip a hand exerciser and press the handles together. Perform three sets of 10 repetitions.

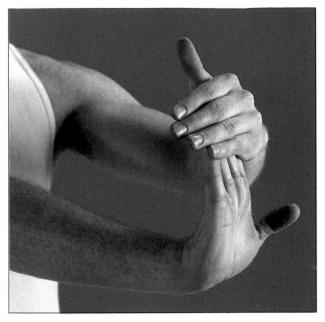

Extend your right arm and open your palm. Pull back gently but firmly on the fingers of your right hand with your left. Hold for 10 seconds; rest and repeat several times for both hands.

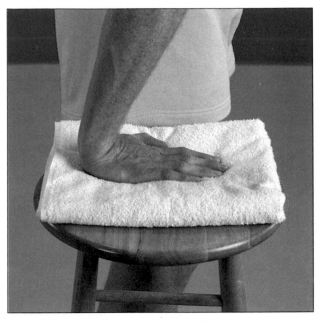

As an alternative to the exercise on the left, stand beside a padded stool and place one palm on it. Lean forwards and hold the stretch for 10 seconds. Repeat with the other hand.

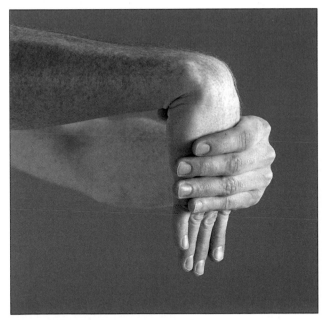

To stretch the forearm muscles that extend your hand, point the fingers of one hand downwards, keeping the wrist straight. With the other hand, press against the knuckles of that hand for at least 10 seconds; switch hands and repeat.

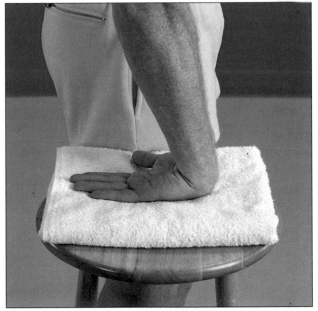

To perform an alternative exercise to the one on the left, place the back of one hand on a padded stool so that the hand and arm form a right angle. Angle your arm backwards and hold for at least 10 seconds. Switch hands and repeat.

101

Wrist and Forearm

Despite its small bones and vulnerable location, the wrist is a relatively sturdy joint because of its network of strong interlocking ligaments and the powerful tendons that run through the area. The wrist is rarely dislocated, but it may be sprained, strained or fractured. This happens when the tendons and muscles of the forearm endure prolonged overuse or when a trauma occurs, such as falling off a horse or slamming into the wall of a squash court at top speed.

The tendons of the muscles in the forearm help to stabilize the wrist and allow it to move. Some of these tendons originate on a bony protuberance on the outside of the elbow. Tendinitis in this area, called tennis elbow, often results from performing backhand strokes with excessive wrist movements, instead of keeping your wrist firm and using the force of your arm and shoulder. Tendinitis in the elbow afflicts not only tennis players, but also anyone who performs repetitive movements with one arm, including golfers, swimmers and carpenters.

To prevent tennis elbow and stress injuries of the wrist and forearm, you should regularly perform the conditioning exercises that are shown on these two pages. Do three sets of 10 repetitions for each exercise.

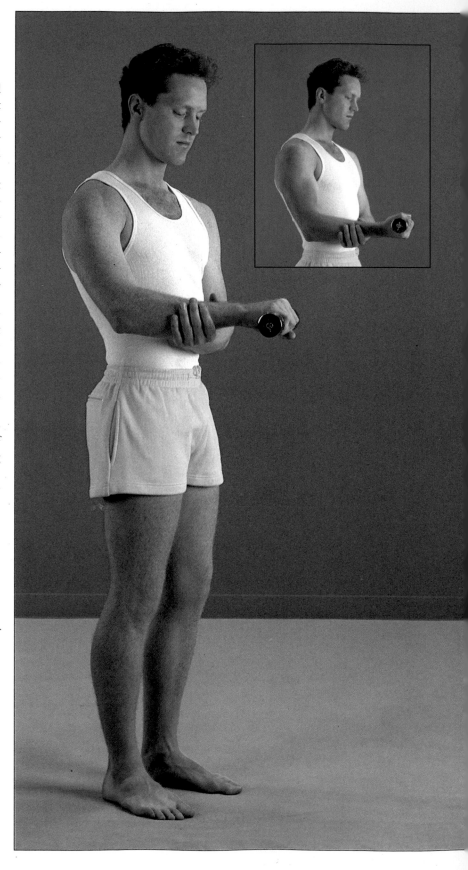

To strengthen the muscles that rotate your wrist, grasp a hand weight in your right hand and use the left to support your right forearm. Rotate your wrist back and forth between the two positions shown above and inset. Change hands and repeat.

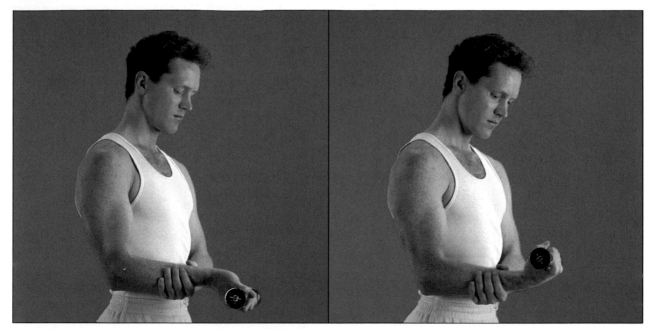

To condition your wrist flexors, grasp a weight in your right hand and support your forearm with your left hand. Alternate between the positions shown above. Change hands and repeat.

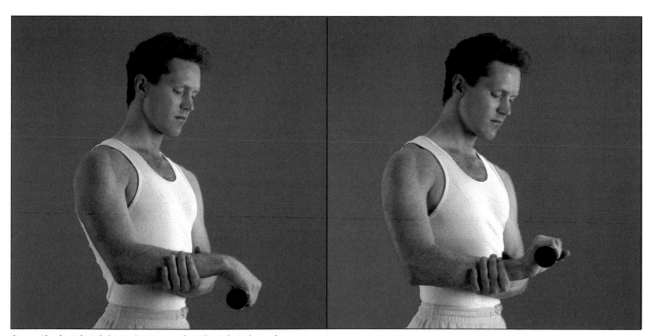

Grasp the hand weight and turn your hand so that the palm faces the floor. Support your forearm with your other hand and alternate between the two positions shown above to strengthen your wrist extensors. Change hands and repeat.

Upper Arm/1

Injuries to the upper arm are relatively rare, but conditioning the muscles in this area is important for maintaining good elbow and shoulder function. The major musculature of the upper arm includes the biceps, a two-part muscle that runs along the front of the arm, bends the elbow and swings the shoulder joint forwards; the brachialis anticus, which bends the elbow and helps it to rotate; and the triceps, a three-part muscle on the back of the arm that acts to straighten the elbow *(see illustration, page 95).*

The exercises shown on these two pages will condition the muscles that extend your elbow, primarily the triceps. The routines on the following two pages will condition the muscles that bend your elbow — the biceps, the brachialis and the brachioradialis. Perform three sets of 10 repetitions of every exercise.

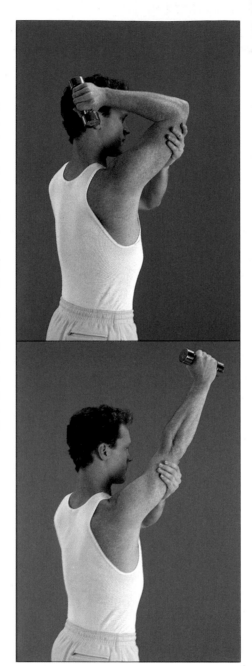

Grasp a hand weight, bend your elbow and raise your upper arm. Support your uplifted arm with your other hand *(top)*. Keep your upper arm in place and extend your elbow *(above)*. Repeat with your other arm.

You can also perform the above exercise with an elastic exercise band. Attach the band to a stationary object behind you, such as a doorknob, so that you feel some tension when you flex your elbow *(right, inset)*. Extend your elbow *(right)*. Repeat for your other arm.

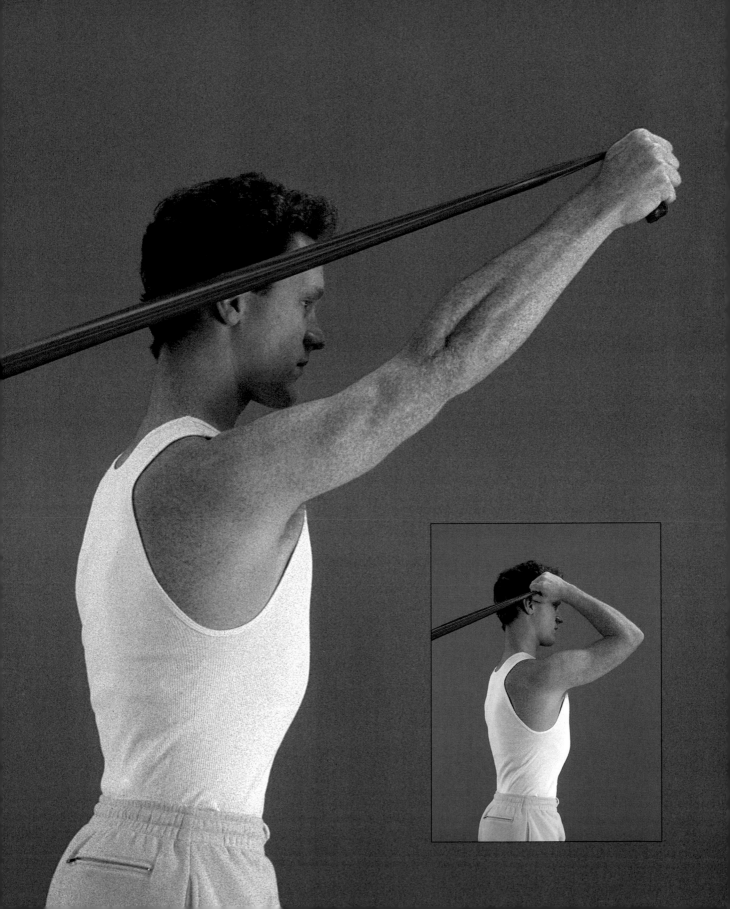

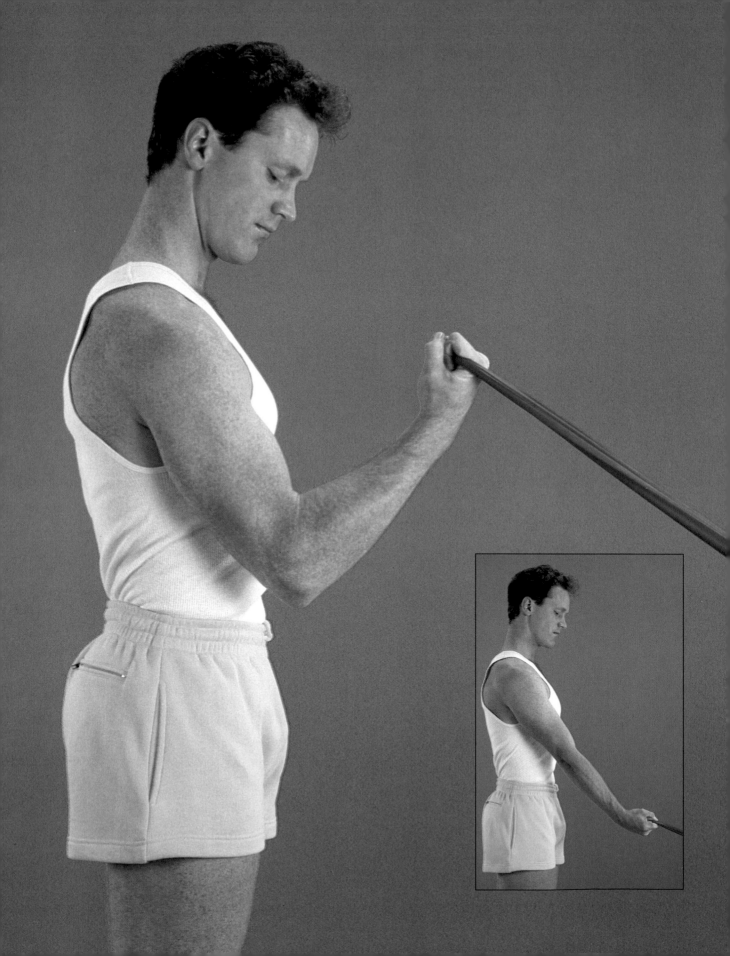

Upper Arm/2

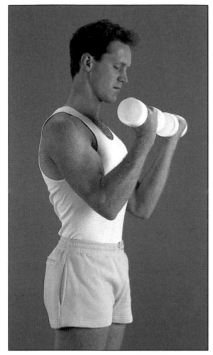

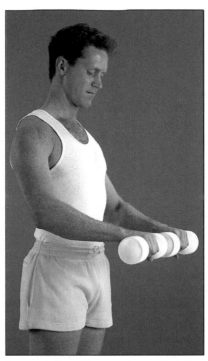

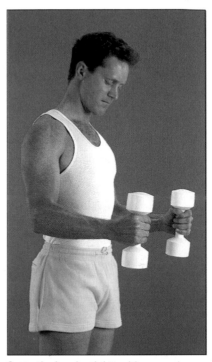

To condition your biceps using hand weights of 1 to 2.5 kilograms, grasp the weights with your palms facing up and bend and extend your elbows.

For a variation of the exercise on the left, to condition the brachialis as well as the biceps, grasp the hand weights with your palms down.

Grasp the hand weights with your palms facing each other. Flex and extend your elbows to condition the brachioradialis and strengthen the elbow flexors.

To condition your biceps with an elastic exercise band, attach the band to a stationary object in front of you so that you feel some tension when you extend your elbow *(opposite, inset)*. Then, keeping your wrist straight, flex your elbow and draw your hand towards your shoulder *(opposite)*. Repeat for your other arm.

Shoulder/1

The flexibility of the shoulder, which allows the joint to swing a full 360 degrees, is crucial to such sports activities as throwing, tennis and swimming; it also enables you to scratch your back and lift a suitcase. This flexibility does, however, have certain drawbacks. The shoulder is the least stable joint in the body. Its socket consists of only a shallow, saucer-like cup and the surrounding ligaments provide little support. As a result, the muscles and tendons that cross the joint provide much of the stability for the shoulder.

Stress injuries to the soft tissues of the shoulder result from repeated use. They can be categorized according to the three shoulder movements involved in throwing and swinging: the cocking phase, the acceleration phase and the follow-through.

Pain in the front of the shoulder as a result of cocking the arm is common among swimmers, gymnasts and tennis and baseball players.

Using your shoulder to "push" a ball may cause stress injuries in the pectoralis major and deltoid muscles or in the tendons.

The acceleration phase of throwing, stroking, lifting or pulling can, in turn, produce stress injuries in the pectoralis major, biceps and triceps.

Stress injuries that result from follow-through can trouble people who play tennis, golf or cricket; in such cases braking muscles along the back of the shoulder, which slow your arm after the ball has been hit or thrown, are affected.

Other common stress injuries to the shoulder include bursitis, or inflammation of the bursal sac in the shoulder joint, and irritated rotator cuff muscles and tendons at the top of the shoulder.

If you are recovering from a shoulder stress injury, the warm-up exercises on these two pages will help you regain mobility. Strengthening and stretching exercises follow on the next six pages.

Place your hands behind your neck, intertwining your fingers, and put your elbows together *(below, left)*. Slowly draw your elbows back as far as you comfortably can *(below)*. Open and close your elbows repeatedly.

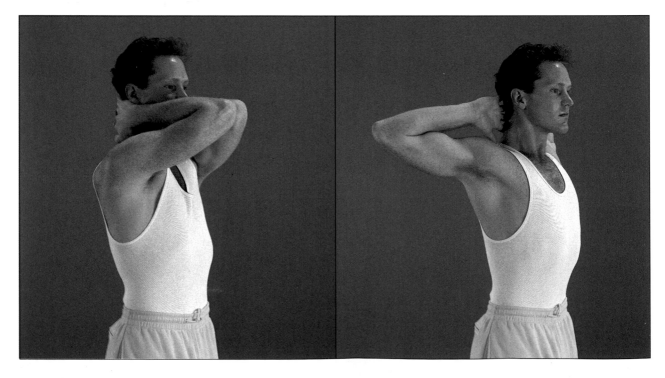

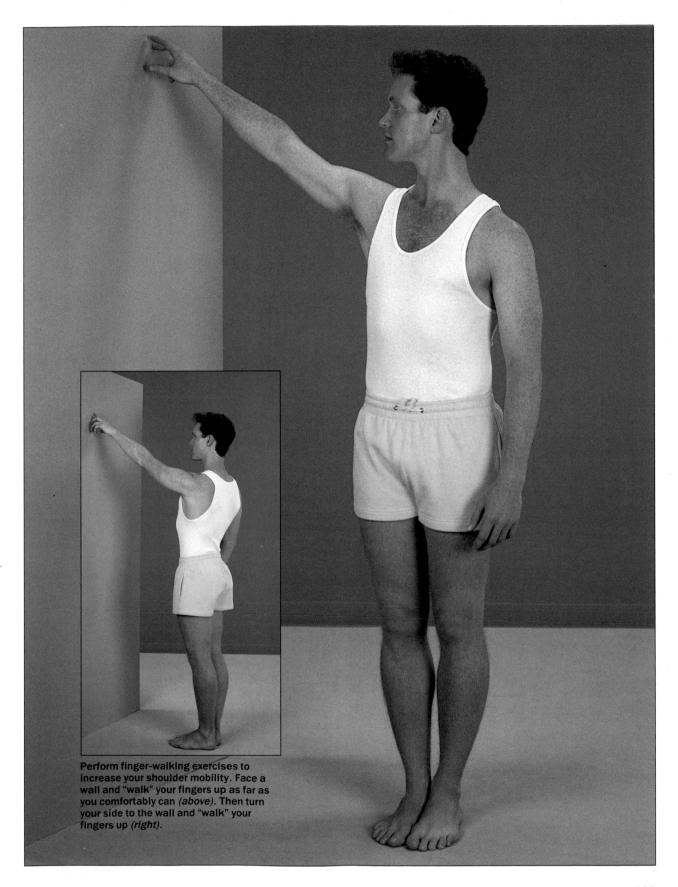

Perform finger-walking exercises to increase your shoulder mobility. Face a wall and "walk" your fingers up as far as you comfortably can *(above)*. Then turn your side to the wall and "walk" your fingers up *(right)*.

Shoulder/2

Use an elastic exercise band to strengthen your shoulder abductors. Stand on the band and hold it so that you feel tension when your hands are at your sides *(right)*. Raise your shoulders towards your ears, then drop your shoulders. Perform three sets of 10 of these shoulder shrugs. Release some of the tension in the band and raise your arms outwards to a level just below shoulder height *(below, right)*. Then perform three sets of 10 forward arm raises *(below)*.

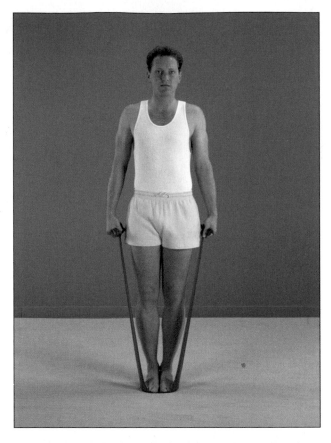

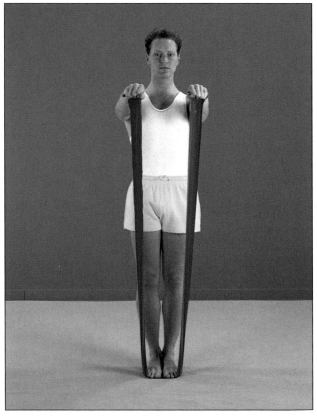

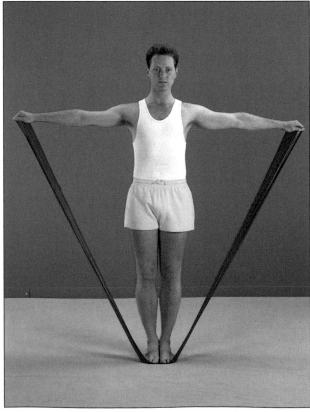

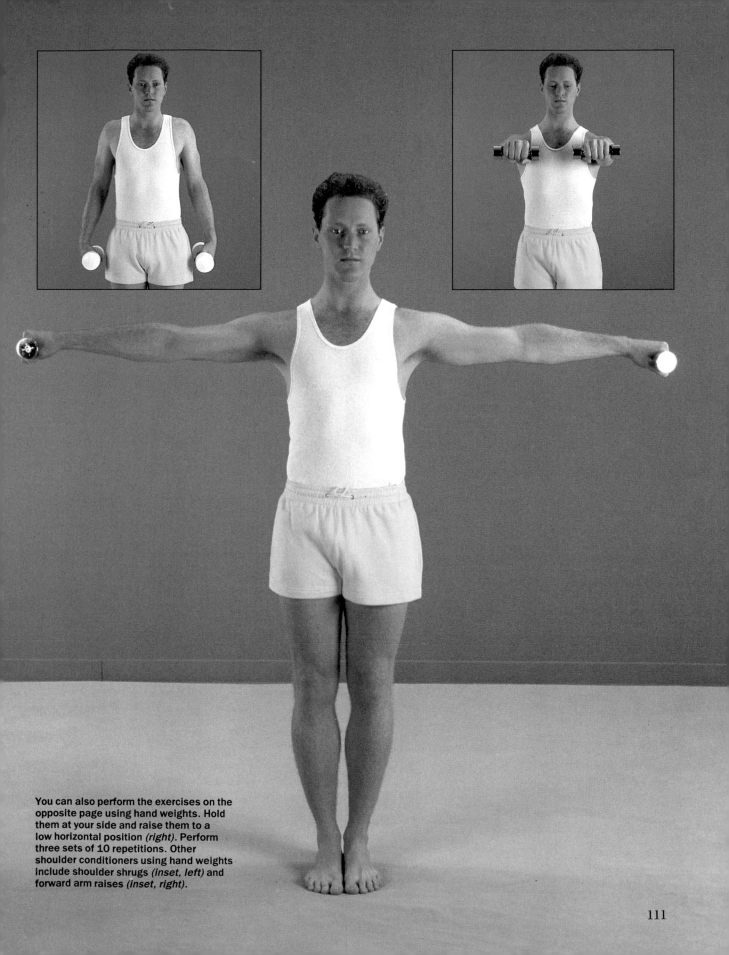

You can also perform the exercises on the opposite page using hand weights. Hold them at your side and raise them to a low horizontal position *(right)*. Perform three sets of 10 repetitions. Other shoulder conditioners using hand weights include shoulder shrugs *(inset, left)* and forward arm raises *(inset, right)*.

Shoulder/3

To perform internal shoulder rotation exercises to strengthen the muscles that turn your arm in towards your body, attach an exercise band to a stationary object such as a doorknob. Stand with your side to the door, grasp the band with your nearer hand and bend your elbow at a right angle *(right)*. Keep your elbow and wrist set and fold your arm across your abdomen *(far right)*. Perform three sets of 10 repetitions, then turn round and repeat for your other arm.

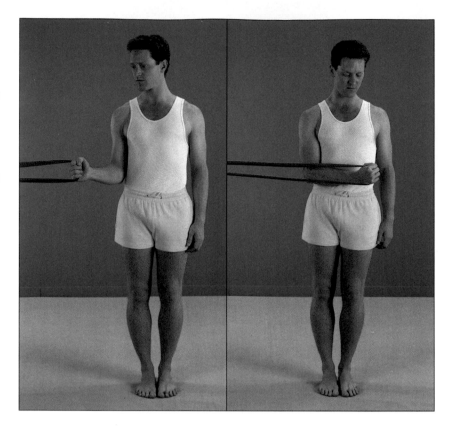

To perform external shoulder rotations to strengthen the muscles that turn your arm away from your body, stand with your side to the door as you did for the internal rotations, but this time grasp the exercise band with the farther arm *(right)*. Keeping your wrist and elbow fixed, swing your arm outwards for three sets of 10 repetitions *(far right)*. Turn round and repeat for your other arm.

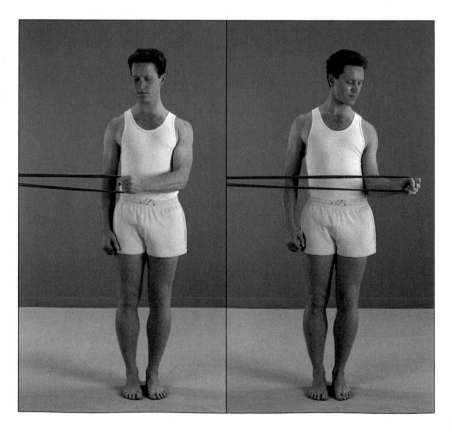

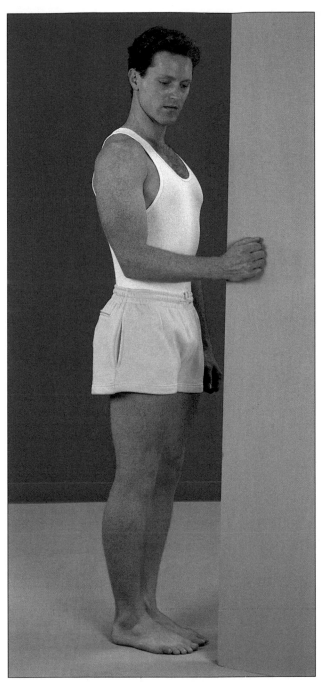

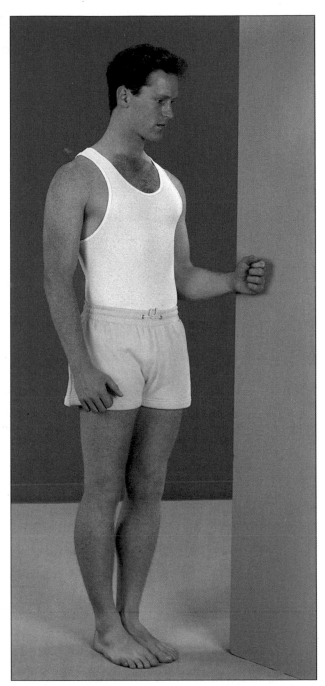

To perform isometric internal rotations without an exercise band, stand at a corner, bend one elbow at a right angle and place your hand, in a loose fist, against the wall. Press as hard as you can for about five seconds. Relax and repeat 10 times for each arm.

To do isometric external rotations, face a corner, bend your elbow at a right angle and place the back of your hand, in a loose fist, against the wall; then press for five seconds. Relax and repeat 10 times. Repeat with the other arm.

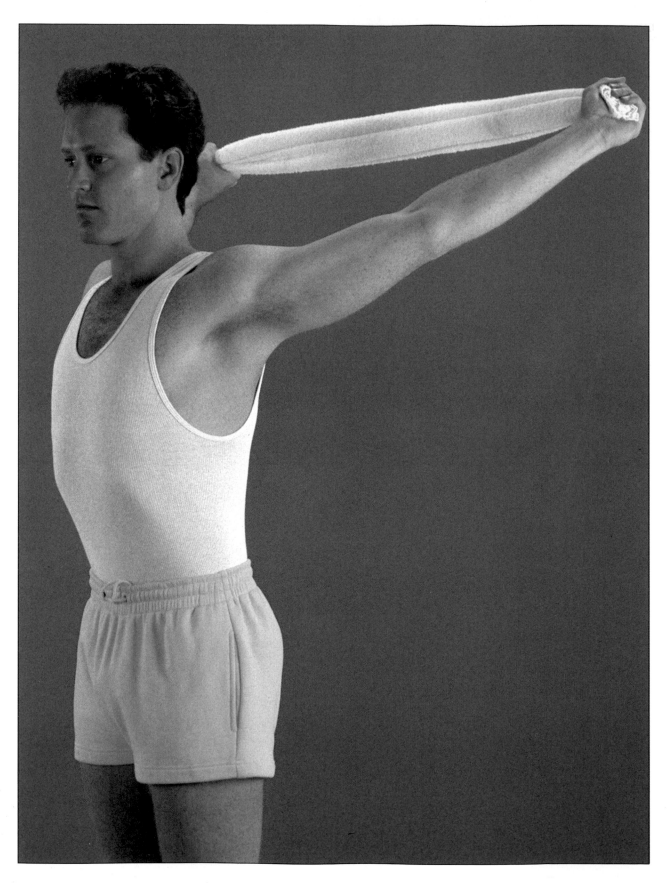

Shoulder/4

Perform an external rotator stretch by holding a towel behind your back and pulling down with the bottom arm, holding for at least 10 seconds. Repeat. Shift arm positions and pull down with your other arm and hold. Repeat.

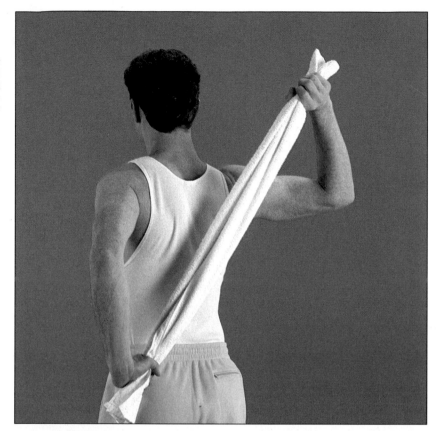

Perform an internal rotator stretch by holding a towel behind your back and pulling up with the raised arm. Reverse arms and repeat.

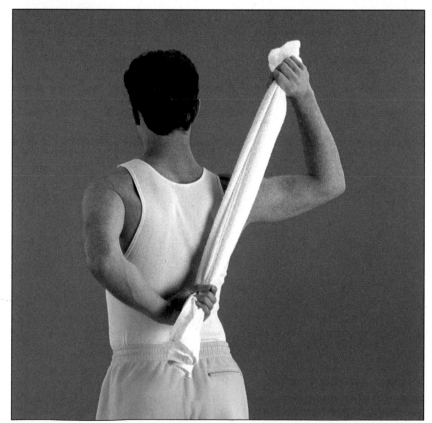

Stand erect with your feet together. Grasp both ends of a towel behind your head (opposite). Hold for at least 10 seconds to stretch your chest, shoulder and upper arm muscles. Repeat at least once.

Back/1

Running down your back from the base of the skull to the pelvis, the spinal column supports and stabilizes the body, acts as a shock absorber and permits movement. Although common, backaches and pains are usually not serious. Many back injuries, however, cause intense pain and can be debilitating. Anyone suffering severe, persistent pain should see a doctor.

Most back injuries affect the lower back, or lumbar spine. Moving up and down or twisting sideways place forces equivalent to several times a person's own body weight on the lower back, which does not have a supplemental support system such as the rib cage. When you arch your back, the spinal column requires increased muscular tension to support itself; the stabilizing muscles can be overstressed. Any activity that also involves lifting an object while you arch your back — even when the weight you lift is your own upper body as you stand up — can place much more stress on the lower back than twisting does.

Most of the muscles that support and move the spine are also attached to it. One exception is the abdominal muscle group in the front of the body. People who experience frequent lower back pain often have weak abdominal muscles. Furthermore, tight hip-flexor muscles can tilt the pelvis forwards and cause excessive curvature of the spine, leading to over-arching. The exercises on this page, and the following five pages, will condition the muscles that support your back. For exercises to increase hip-flexor flexibility, turn to pages 82-83.

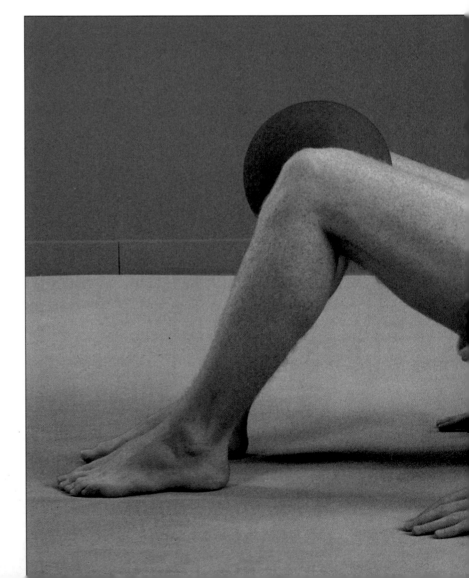

To improve your spinal strength and mobility, lie on your back, bend your knees and place your feet flat on the floor. Grip a ball firmly between your knees; raise your pelvis off the floor and then gently lower it. Repeat as many times as you can.

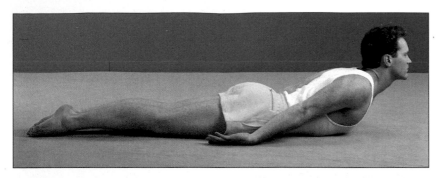

To strengthen your back extensor muscles, the muscles that prevent you from slouching, lie face down on the floor with your arms at your sides. Lift your head and chest off the ground as high as you can, hold for five seconds, then rest. Gradually increase to 10 seconds.

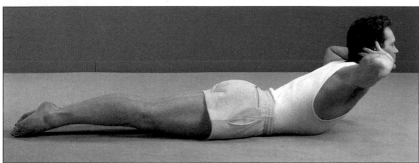

As the strength of your back extensors improves, you can increase the difficulty of this exercise by placing your hands behind your head. Lift your chest off the floor and hold for no more than five seconds, then rest. Work up to three sets of 10 repetitions.

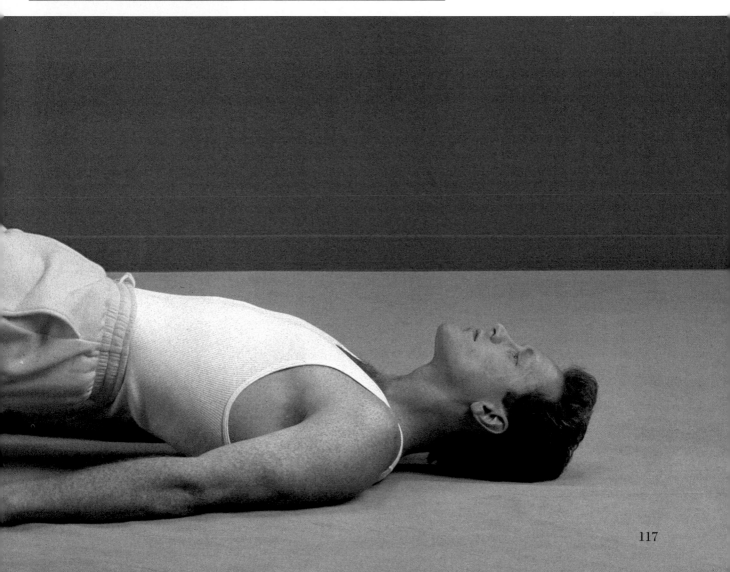

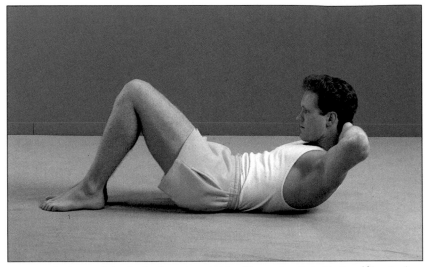

To strengthen your abdominals, lie on your back with your hands behind your head and your knees bent. Curl up so that your shoulder blades are off the floor, then slowly curl back down. Start slowly and increase the number of repetitions daily.

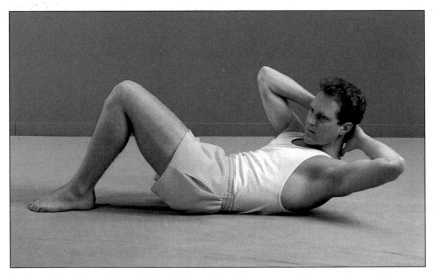

To strengthen your oblique abdominals, perform the same curl-up exercise as shown above but twist slightly to the side. Alternate twisting right and left.

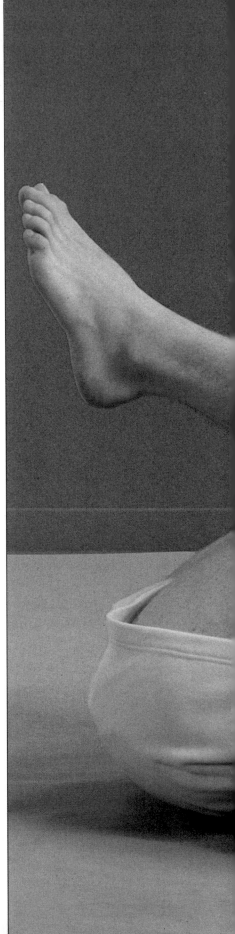

To stretch your lower back, lie on your back, grasp your thighs behind your knees and draw your knees towards your chest *(right)*. Hold for no more than five seconds, relax and repeat five to 10 times. As a variation you can draw one knee to your chest at a time *(inset)*.

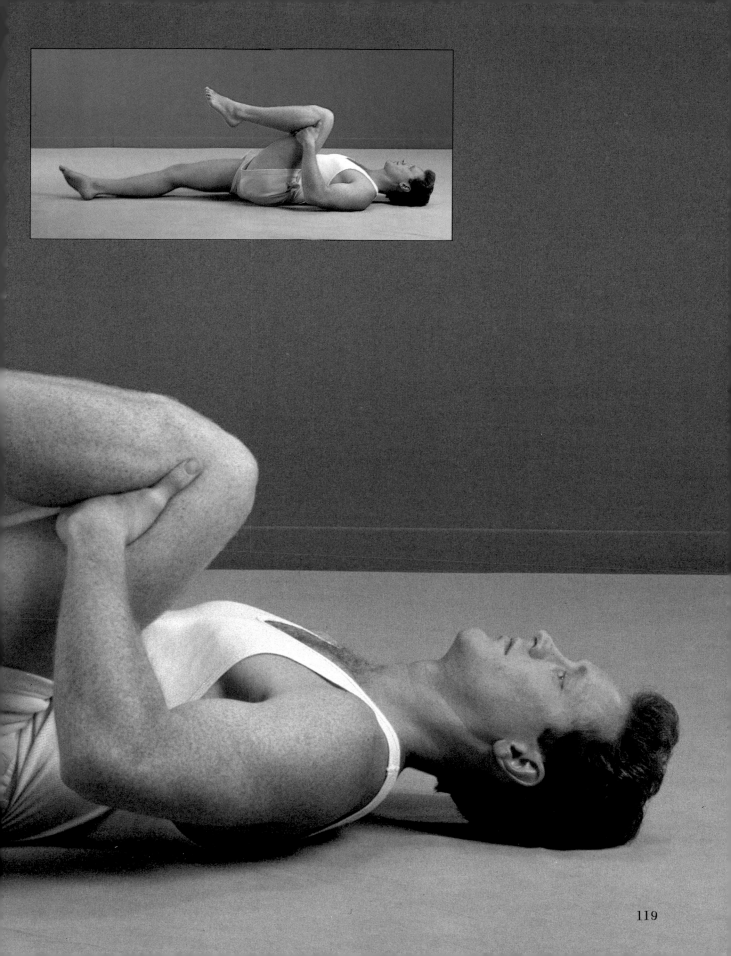

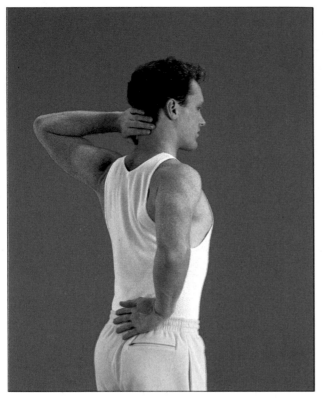

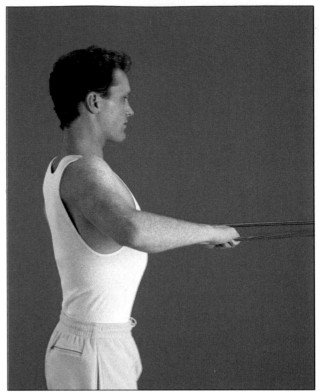

Place one hand on the small of your back and the other behind your neck. This will pull your shoulders back and draw your shoulder blades together, strengthening the muscles that enhance posture. Hold for 10 seconds, switch sides and repeat.

Attach an exercise band to a doorknob or other stationary object to perform another exercise for the shoulder blades, known as a scapular retraction. Grasp the band with both hands and pull it back, drawing your shoulder blades together.

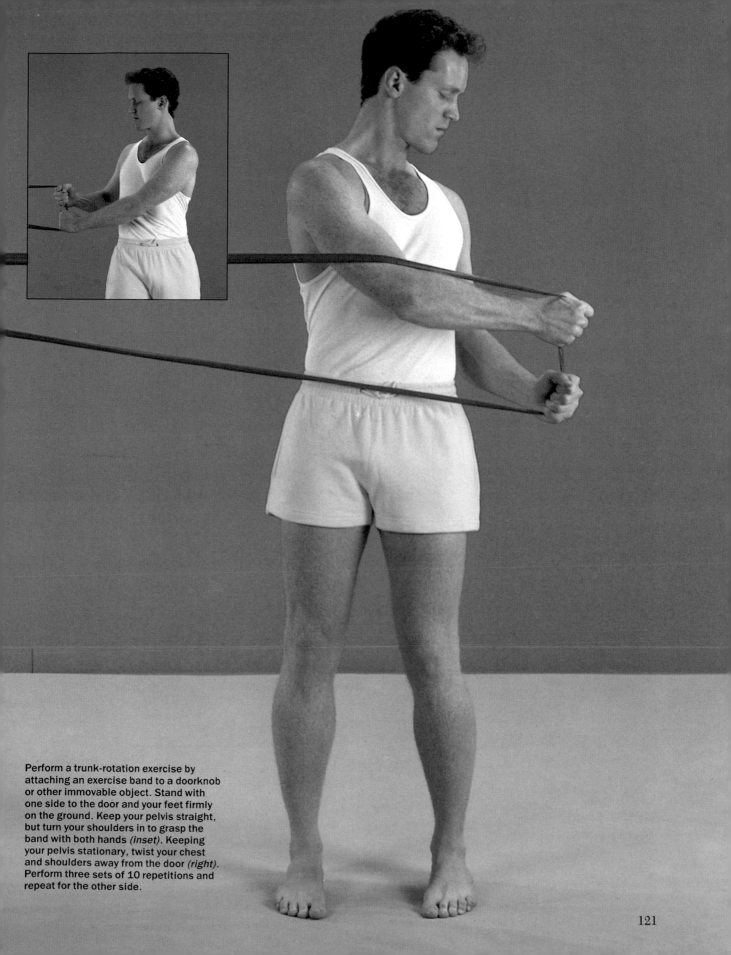

Perform a trunk-rotation exercise by attaching an exercise band to a doorknob or other immovable object. Stand with one side to the door and your feet firmly on the ground. Keep your pelvis straight, but turn your shoulders in to grasp the band with both hands *(inset)*. Keeping your pelvis stationary, twist your chest and shoulders away from the door *(right)*. Perform three sets of 10 repetitions and repeat for the other side.

Neck

The most flexible part of your spine, the neck is comprised of seven vertebrae that allow your head to rotate virtually 180 degrees. You can also flex your neck to allow your chin to touch your chest, extend your neck to look upwards, and flex laterally so that your ear can drop towards your shoulder.

Stiffness is the most common neck complaint, and, unlike other upper body aches and pains, it is not always caused by overexertion. For instance, the wrong sleeping position can sometimes result in neck stiffness. You can best treat this particular stiffness by stretching the neck in the direction opposite the tightness. If your stiff neck tilts your head to the left, for example, slowly tilt your head to the right.

You can help to prevent neck stiffness by improving the strength and flexibility of your neck muscles. Turn your head left, hold for five to 10 seconds and then turn to the right and hold. Drop your chin to your chest and hold for five to 10 seconds.

Tilt your left ear towards your left shoulder and then your right ear to your right shoulder, each for five to 10 seconds. In order to condition your neck muscles further, perform the routines that are demonstrated on these two pages.

A heavy blow to the head or neck region can cause a serious — even fatal — injury. If you suspect that someone has received such an injury, make him as comfortable as possible but do not move him. Get medical attention immediately.

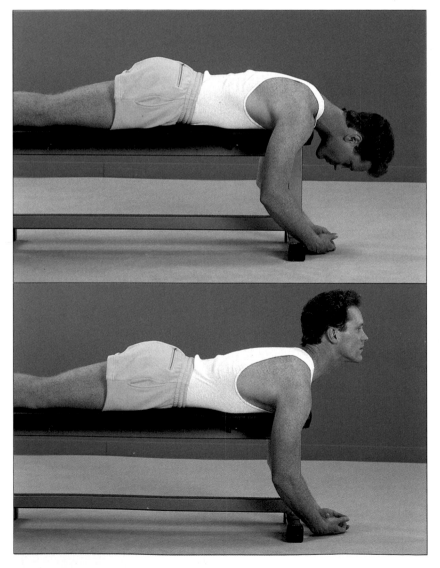

Lie face down on an exercise table with your arms dangling loosely and your head extended over the edge of the table *(left, top)*. Raise your head up slowly *(left)* and return it to the starting position. Be sure not to jerk your head. Perform three sets of 10 repetitions to strengthen your neck extensors, the muscles that draw your head back.

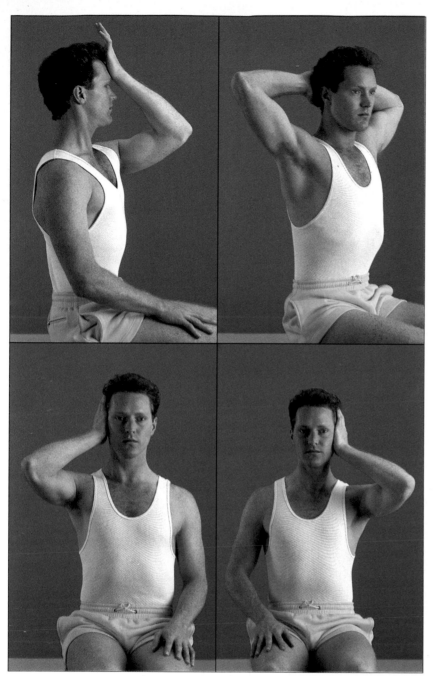

Perform isometric exercises to improve your neck strength. Do each exercise for five seconds and repeat 10 times. Clockwise from far left: sit in a chair with your back straight and place one palm against your forehead. Press your head forwards while you resist its movement with your hand. Next, interlace your fingers behind your head to resist movement as you push your head back. Then place your left hand against the left side of your head and push your head against your hand's resistance. Finally, repeat the exercise with the right side of your head pushing against your right hand's resistance.

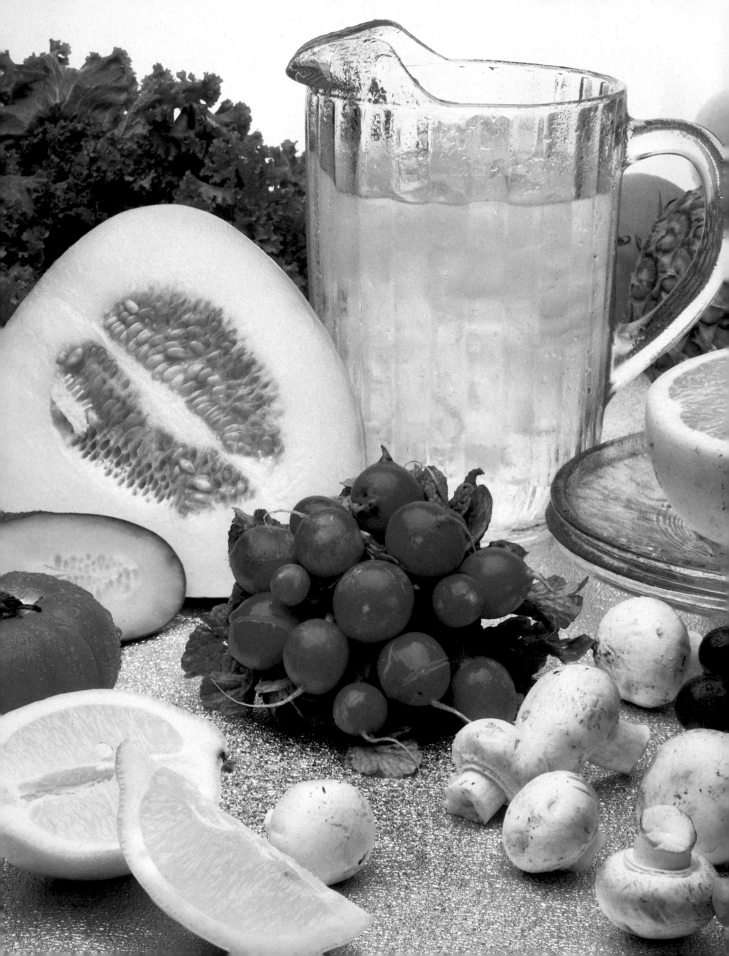

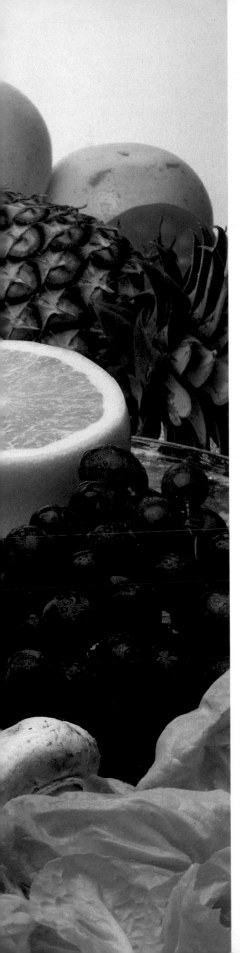

CHAPTER FIVE

Fluids

Crucial benefits, the best ways to replace fluids lost during exercise

Of all the nutrients that you consume, the one most crucial to your survival is water. While it is possible to survive without food for weeks, you can live for only a few days without restoring your body's supply of water. Ordinarily you lose an average of two to three litres of water daily from excretions, perspiration and the water vapour you exhale. When you exercise, however, particularly in hot weather, your rate of fluid loss through perspiration increases dramatically.

A person exercising at a moderate to high level of intensity on a hot day may lose two litres of water or more over three to four hours. If you do not drink enough water to make up for the fluid you lose while working out, your speed, endurance and strength may suffer. Studies of athletes show that a deficit of water equal to just 2 per cent of body weight can slow blood circulation and diminish concentration. Drinking too little water during exercise can also lead to dizziness, nausea

125

and cramps. And during prolonged periods of exertion, inadequate fluid replacement can produce such severe dehydration that you lose the ability to perspire. In extreme cases, the accompanying rise in internal body temperature can lead to heat stroke, which can be fatal.

Apart from its role in maintaining your body's temperature, water functions as the main solvent and transport medium within the body. It dissolves food and carries the nutrients, hormones and oxygen from one part of your body to another in blood plasma.

The water inside your body contains dissolved minerals known as electrolytes, which are electrically charged particles that control and maintain the proper balance between the water inside the body's cells and the water surrounding them. The most important electrolytes are potassium, sodium, calcium, magnesium and chloride.

The abundance of salt — comprised of sodium and chloride — in the average diet usually compensates for the sodium and chloride lost in perspiration. However, potassium and magnesium, which are in most fruits and vegetables, and calcium, found in dairy products and some vegetables, may be lacking in some diets. These three electrolytes are crucial for muscle functions and for the cardiovascular system. Apart from its role in bone development and strength, calcium aids the contraction and relaxation of your muscles. Potassium enables your muscles to use carbohydrates for energy. Magnesium also takes part in the muscles' energy production, conducts nerve impulses to and from the spine and contributes to normal muscle functions. Recent research suggests that some of these electrolytes are also necessary for preventing elevated blood pressure and keeping your heart beating properly; they may also protect you against strokes.

Because fruits and vegetables are high in water and have an abundance of electrolytes, they are particularly important components of your diet when you exercise. Some types of lettuce contain 95 per cent water, for example, while raw carrots and oranges are 85 to 90 per cent water. Almost all the recipes in this chapter provide generous amounts of these mineral-rich, low-sodium foods. For instance, the Pear and Endive Salad on page 136 and the Plum-Cantaloupe Salad on page 137 contain electrolytes, other minerals and water.

A diet that includes adequate amounts of fruit and vegetables will keep you well supplied with potassium and magnesium. If you want to replenish these supplies after a workout, choose an unsweetened fruit juice. Research on endurance athletes has shown that drinks containing small amounts of sugar can improve performance in long-distance events such as the marathon, but sugary drinks — including commercial soft drinks — do not provide significant help during shorter events. Nor is drinking coffee or tea a good way in which to replace lost water: both of these beverages act as diuretics and therefore actually increase water loss. Studies have repeatedly confirmed that drinking plenty of plain water is the best way to replace the water that is lost during most forms of exercise.

W HEN YOU EXERCISE

Drink plain cool water. Studies show that your body absorbs water best when chilled to 5 to 10°C.

Drink at least one 25 centilitre glass of water just before you begin to exercise.

Drink a glass of water every 15 to 20 minutes while you exercise.

Drink more water than you think you need. You can easily quench your thirst before you have replaced all the water you have lost while exercising.

Drink 25 to 50 centilitres of water after you have finished.

The Basic Guidelines

For a moderately active adult, Britain's National Advisory Committee on Nutrition Education recommends a diet that is low in fat, high in carbohydrates and moderate in protein. The committee's proposals for the long term suggest that no more than 30 per cent of your calories come from fat, that around 11 per cent come from protein and hence that 55 to 60 per cent come from carbohydrates. A gram of fat equals nine calories, while a gram of protein or carbohydrate equals four calories; therefore, if you eat 2,100 calories a day, you should consume approximately 70 grams of fat, 310 grams of carbohydrate and 60 grams of protein daily. If you follow a low-fat/high-carbohydrate diet, your chance of developing heart disease, cancer and other life-threatening diseases may be considerably reduced.

◆ The nutrition charts that accompany each of the low-fat/high-carbohydrate recipes in this book include the number of calories per serving, the number of grams of fat, carbohydrate and protein in a serving, and the percentage of calories derived from each of these nutrients. In addition, the charts provide the amount of calcium, iron and sodium per serving.

◆ Calcium deficiency may be associated with periodontal diseases — which attack the mouth's bones and tissues, including the gums — in both men and women, and with osteoporosis, or bone shrinking and weakening, in elderly women. The deficiency may also contribute to high blood pressure. The daily allowance for calcium recommended by the United Kingdom Department of Health and Social Security (DHSS) is 500 milligrams a day for men and women. Pregnant and lactating women are advised to consume 1,200 milligrams daily.

◆ Although one way you can reduce your fat intake is to cut your consumption of red meat, you should make sure that you get your necessary iron from other sources. The DHSS suggests a minimum of 10 milligrams of iron per day for men and 12 milligrams for women between the ages of 18 and 54.

◆ High sodium intake is associated with high blood pressure in susceptible people. Most adults should restrict sodium intake to about 2,000 milligrams a day, according to the World Health Organization. One way to keep sodium consumption in check is not to add table salt to food.

Contrary to popular belief, consuming salt tablets during or after exercise is not only unnecessary but can be dangerous. The average person already consumes more than enough salt to supply bodily needs, even during exercise in warm weather. Since your stomach draws water away from the rest of the body in order to absorb salt, taking these tablets when you are dehydrated worsens the condition.

The following recipes present soups, salads and desserts, as well as drinks. Consuming these foods and drinks, in conjunction with other fruits and vegetables, will generally supply you with sufficient electrolytes to make sports drinks or mineral supplements unnecessary. Of course, whenever you work out, and especially in hot water, you should ensure that you drink plenty of cool water before, during and after exercising *(see box, opposite)*.

Breakfast

FRUIT KEBABS WITH COCONUT SAUCE

If you eat these kebabs instead of drinking fruit juice at breakfast, you will benefit from cholesterol-lowering fibre and fulfil your vitamin C requirement, too.

CALORIES per serving	125
73% Carbohydrate	26 g
15% Protein	5 g
12% Fat	2 g
CALCIUM	52 mg
IRON	1 mg
SODIUM	128 mg

125 g (4 oz) low-fat cottage cheese (1% fat)

2 tablespoons low-fat vanilla yogurt

2 tablespoons sweetened flaked coconut

1 tablespoon sugar

300 g (10 oz) strawberries, washed

175 g (6 oz) black grapes, washed and stemmed

½ large pineapple, halved lengthwise and cut into 1 cm (½ inch) thick triangles

For the sauce, combine the cottage cheese, yogurt, coconut and sugar in a food processor or blender and process until smooth, scraping down the sides of the container with a rubber spatula. Transfer the sauce to a small bowl. Thread the strawberries, grapes and pineapple pieces alternately on each of eight bamboo skewers and serve with the coconut sauce.   Makes 4 servings

Fruit Kebabs with Coconut Sauce

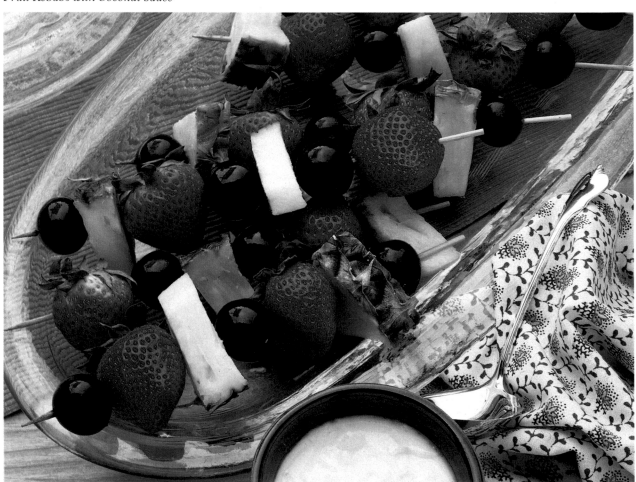

RAISIN BRAN-BANANA SHAKE

When you have this shake for breakfast, you increase your fluid intake while getting plenty of potassium from the yogurt, banana and raisins. Wheat bran, a good source of iron, also contains magnesium, which recent studies suggest may help prevent high blood pressure.

25 cl (8 fl oz) plain low-fat yogurt
1 banana, peeled, frozen and cut into large chunks
45 g (1½ oz) raisins

30 g (1 oz) coarsely chopped unpeeled Golden Delicious apple
1 tablespoon wheat bran

CALORIES per serving	380
76% Carbohydrate	78 g
14% Protein	15 g
10% Fat	5 g
CALCIUM	446 mg
IRON	2 mg
SODIUM	165 mg

Combine all the ingredients in a food processor or blender and process until blended. Pour the shake into a tall glass and serve.   Makes 1 serving

BANANA HOT CHOCOLATE

Skimmed milk forms the basis for this hot chocolate drink, which is a low-fat, complete breakfast.

15 g (½ oz) plain chocolate
12.5 cl (4 fl oz) skimmed milk
1 teaspoon pure maple syrup

1 teaspoon decaffeinated instant coffee granules
1 banana, peeled

CALORIES per serving	240
71% Carbohydrate	45 g
9% Protein	6 g
20% Fat	6 g
CALCIUM	171 mg
IRON	1 mg
SODIUM	67 mg

Combine the chocolate with 2 tablespoons of water in a small saucepan and heat over very low heat, stirring constantly, until the chocolate is melted. Add another 6 tablespoons of water, the milk, maple syrup and coffee granules. Increase the heat to medium and heat the mixture for 5 to 7 minutes, or until it is hot. Meanwhile, purée the banana in a food processor or blender. Gradually pour in the hot chocolate milk mixture and continue processing until blended. Pour the hot chocolate into a large mug and serve.   Makes 1 serving

KIWI-LIME SHAKE

Kiwi fruit, higher in vitamin C than citrus fruit, flavours this unusual shake, and low-fat ricotta cheese thickens it. Thirst-quenching as well as nutritionally balanced, this is a good all-in-one breakfast to have after a morning workout.

2 kiwi fruits
1 banana
1 teaspoon lime juice
½ teaspoon grated lime rind

2 ice cubes
25 cl (8 fl oz) skimmed milk
60 g (2 oz) low-fat ricotta cheese

CALORIES per serving	185
67% Carbohydrate	32 g
18% Protein	9 g
15% Fat	3 g
CALCIUM	259 mg
IRON	1 mg
SODIUM	107 mg

Peel the kiwi fruits and the banana and cut them into large chunks. Place the fruit, lime juice, lime rind and ice cubes in a food processor or blender and process until blended. Add the milk and ricotta and process for another 5 to 10 seconds, scraping down the sides of the container with a rubber spatula. Pour the shake into two tall glasses and serve immediately.   Makes 2 servings

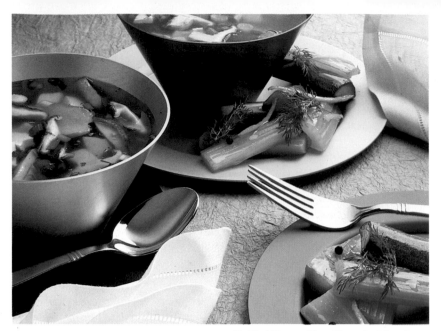

Pickled Vegetables, Shiitake Miso Soup

Lunch

PICKLED VEGETABLES

A serving of this side dish provides more than your recommended daily intake of vitamin A, essential for healthy skin. The vegetables are much lower in sodium than most commercially bottled pickles, and they contain virtually no fat, making them a good lunchtime substitute for crisps or corn chips.

CALORIES per serving	60
84% Carbohydrate	14 g
12% Protein	2 g
4% Fat	0.3 g
CALCIUM	87 mg
IRON	2 mg
SODIUM	210 mg

250 g (8 oz) carrots
250 g (8 oz) courgettes
250 g (8 oz) celery
¼ teaspoon salt, approximately
12.5 cl (4 fl oz) herb vinegar or red wine vinegar

1 tablespoon sugar, or less to taste
1 teaspoon whole peppercorns
1 teaspoon finely julienned lemon rind
3 small garlic cloves
10 dill sprigs

Scrub and trim the carrots and courgettes, halve them lengthwise and cut them into 5 cm (2 inch) pieces. Trim the celery and cut it into 5 cm (2 inch) strips. Bring a large saucepan of water to the boil over high heat and add a pinch of salt. Add the carrots, reduce the heat to medium and cook for 3 to 4 minutes, then increase the heat to high. When the water returns to the boil, add the courgettes and celery, and cook for 1 minute. Drain the vegetables in a colander, cool them under cold running water until well chilled and drain again. Transfer to a large bowl or storage jar. Add the vinegar, sugar, peppercorns, lemon rind, garlic, dill and ¼ teaspoon of salt, and toss to combine. Cover the bowl and refrigerate overnight, stirring the mixture occasionally. Serve the vegetables chilled or at room temperature. They will keep for 3 to 4 days in a covered container in the refrigerator. Makes 4 servings

SHIITAKE MISO SOUP

Packaged miso soup mixes are convenient but often loaded with sodium in the form of the flavour enhancer MSG (monosodium glutamate). Low-sodium chicken stock and light miso are used here to keep the sodium level low.

CALORIES per serving	50
51% Carbohydrate	7 g
23% Protein	3 g
26% Fat	1 g
CALCIUM	34 mg
IRON	1 mg
SODIUM	191 mg

25 cl (8 fl oz) low-sodium chicken
    stock (see page 134)
125 g (4 oz) fresh shiitake
    mushrooms, trimmed and sliced
    5 mm (¼ inch) thick
60 g (2 oz) tofu, diced
2 tablespoons light miso

3 slices fresh ginger root
¼ teaspoon sesame oil
30 g (1 oz) spring onions,
    coarsely chopped
1 tablespoon chopped fresh
    coriander

Combine the stock with 75 cl (1 ¼ pints) of water in a medium-sized saucepan and bring to the boil over medium heat. Stir in the mushrooms, tofu, miso, ginger and sesame oil, reduce the heat to low and simmer the soup for 10 minutes. Remove the pan from the heat and stir in the spring onions and coriander. Ladle the soup into four bowls and serve.   Makes 4 servings

Note: if fresh shiitake mushrooms are unavailable, substitute fresh button mushrooms. Miso is a fermented soya bean paste used as a seasoning and soup base in Japanese cooking. The light-coloured *shiromiso*, made with rice, is milder and less salty than the reddish-brown *akamiso*, made with barley.

CARROT AND LEEK SOUP

Vegetable soups — and vegetables themselves — are good sources of water. Carrots, for instance, are 90 per cent water, and in addition they provide vitamin A in the form of beta carotene.

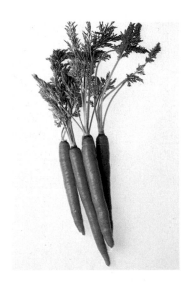

250 g (8 oz) leeks
2 garlic cloves, crushed
15 g (½ oz) butter or margarine
500 g (1 lb) carrots, trimmed and
    cut into 5 cm (2 inch) pieces

250 g (8 oz) potatoes, peeled
    and quartered
50 cl (16 fl oz) low-sodium
    chicken stock (see page 134)
4 tablespoons chopped fresh dill
¼ teaspoon pepper

CALORIES per serving	150
70% Carbohydrate	27 g
8% Protein	3 g
22% Fat	4 g
CALCIUM	72 mg
IRON	2 mg
SODIUM	80 mg

Trim the leeks, split them lengthwise and wash them carefully under cold running water to remove any grit and sand. Cut the leeks into 5 cm (2 inch) pieces. Place the leeks, garlic and butter in a medium-sized saucepan, cover and cook over low heat for 5 minutes. Add the carrots, potatoes, stock, dill, pepper and 25 cl (8 fl oz) of water, increase the heat to medium high and bring the mixture to the boil. Cover the pan, reduce the heat to low and simmer the soup for 15 to 20 minutes, or until the potatoes are tender. Remove the pan from the heat, uncover it and allow the soup to cool for 20 minutes. Transfer the soup to a food processor or blender and process until smooth, then return it to the pan and reheat for 5 to 10 minutes over medium heat. Ladle the soup into four bowls and serve.   Makes 4 servings

CREAMY CUCUMBER SOUP

CALORIES per serving	100
65% Carbohydrate	17 g
23% Protein	6 g
12% Fat	1 g
CALCIUM	207 mg
IRON	1 mg
SODIUM	251 mg

Buttermilk is made from skimmed or semi-skimmed milk and has only about 1 gram of fat per 25 cl (8 fl oz). Generally, low-fat foods are quickly digested, so you can exercise shortly after eating them without fear of an upset stomach.

500 g (1 lb) cucumbers
1 onion
2 slices fresh ginger root
12.5 cl (4 fl oz) vegetable stock (see page 134)

25 cl (8 fl oz) buttermilk
2 tablespoons chopped fresh dill
¼ teaspoon pepper
Pinch of salt

Peel and trim the cucumbers, halve them lengthwise and scoop out the seeds with a teaspoon. Cut the cucumbers crosswise into 3 mm (⅛ inch) thick slices. Peel the onion and cut it into thin wedges. Combine the cucumbers, onion and ginger in a medium-sized saucepan, add the stock and 12.5 cl (4 fl oz) of water and bring to the boil over medium heat. Reduce the heat to low, cover the pan and simmer for 30 minutes. Stir in the buttermilk, dill, pepper and salt; transfer the soup to a food processor or blender and process until puréed. Serve the soup hot, or let it cool to room temperature, refrigerate it for about 4 hours and serve it very cold. Makes 2 servings

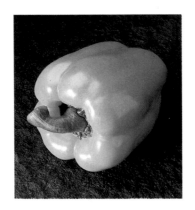

PEPPER PARSNIP SOUP

Parsnips are a good source of potassium, a mineral required for proper functioning of the muscles, including the heart.

2 sweet yellow peppers, seeded and cut into chunks
2 parsnips, cut into chunks
1 onion, sliced
2 garlic cloves, crushed

50 cl (16 fl oz) low-sodium chicken stock (see page 134)
1 tablespoon chopped fresh chives, plus additional chives for garnish (optional)
¼ teaspoon pepper

CALORIES per serving	75
81% Carbohydrate	16 g
8% Protein	2 g
11% Fat	1 g
CALCIUM	34 mg
IRON	1 mg
SODIUM	12 mg

Place the sweet peppers, parsnips, onion, garlic, stock, chopped chives, pepper and 25 cl (8 fl oz) of water in a medium-sized saucepan and bring to the boil over medium-high heat. Cover the pan, reduce the heat to low and simmer the vegetables for 25 to 30 minutes. Remove the pan from the heat, uncover it and allow the soup to cool for 30 minutes. Transfer the soup to a food processor or blender and process until blended. Reheat the soup briefly over medium heat and serve hot, or cool it to room temperature, then cover and refrigerate it for 3 to 4 hours and serve it chilled. Ladle the soup into four bowls and garnish with additional chives if desired. Makes 4 servings

Dinner

HERBED GAZPACHO

Gazpacho, often called a liquid salad, is traditionally thickened with oil and breadcrumbs, but this version is lighter and more refreshing. Tomatoes, the main ingredient, contain both vitamin C and iron; vitamin C aids in the body's absorption of iron.

CALORIES per serving	60
76% Carbohydrate	13 g
16% Protein	3 g
8% Fat	1 g
CALCIUM	99 mg
IRON	2 mg
SODIUM	380 mg

850 g (28 oz) canned plum tomatoes, with their liquid
250 g (8 oz) unpeeled cucumber, finely chopped
45 g (1½ oz) spring onions, finely chopped
45 g (1½ oz) celery, finely diced

4 tablespoons chopped fresh basil
2 tablespoons herb vinegar or red wine vinegar
1 small garlic clove, crushed
½ teaspoon pepper
Pinch of salt

Combine the tomatoes and their liquid with all the remaining ingredients in a large bowl; stir well to break up the tomatoes. Cover the bowl and refrigerate the gazpacho for 4 hours, or until thoroughly chilled. Stir the soup to reblend it before serving and serve it over ice cubes, if desired.   Makes 4 servings

Herbed Gazpacho

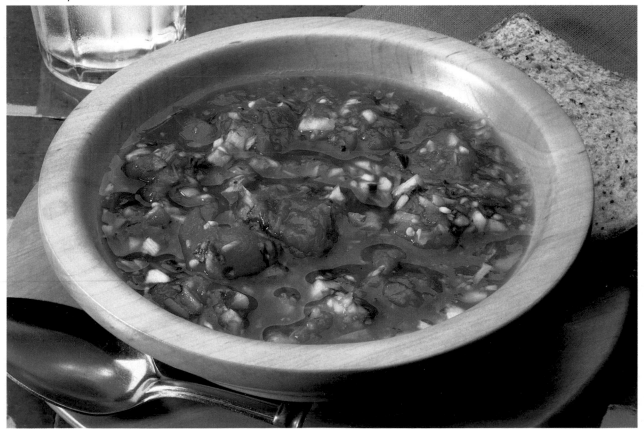

VEGETABLE STOCK

Home-made stock, a kitchen staple for healthy cooking, is easy to prepare. Freeze 25 cl (8 fl oz) portions of this nearly fat-free stock, then just add seasonal produce and other fresh ingredients to make nourishing soups.

CALORIES per 25 cl (8 fl oz)	25
87% Carbohydrate	6 g
10% Protein	1 g
3% Fat	0.1 g
CALCIUM	27 mg
IRON	1 mg
SODIUM	169 mg

500 g (1 lb) green cabbage	1 unpeeled garlic clove
250 g (8 oz) leeks	6 parsley sprigs
125 g (4 oz) parsnips	½ teaspoon salt
1 large carrot	½ teaspoon whole peppercorns
1 stick celery	

Core and coarsely chop the cabbage. Trim the leeks, split them lengthwise and wash them carefully under cold running water to remove any grit and sand. Coarsely chop the leeks. Wash, trim and halve the parsnips, carrot and celery. Place the vegetables in a stockpot, add the garlic, parsley, salt, peppercorns and 2 litres (3½ pints) of water, and bring to the boil over medium-high heat. Reduce the heat to medium low, cover the pot and simmer for 1 hour. Uncover the pot and simmer the stock for another 45 minutes.

Strain the stock through a colander set over a large bowl; discard the solids. Transfer the stock to storage jars or containers and refrigerate or freeze it. The stock will keep for up to a week in the refrigerator, but it should be heated to a boil for 5 minutes after 2 to 3 days, then cooled and returned to the refrigerator. The stock may be frozen for 1 month.   Makes 1.75 litres (3 pints)

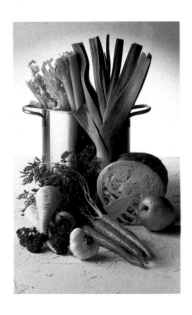

LOW-SODIUM CHICKEN STOCK

Making your own chicken stock is the best way to control its salt content. Stock cubes have as many as 850 milligrams of sodium per 25 cl (8 fl oz) serving.

500 g (1 lb) raw chicken bones, such as necks or backs	1 stick celery, halved
	1 unpeeled garlic clove
2 large carrots, halved	1 bay leaf
1 onion, unpeeled	4 whole peppercorns

CALORIES per 25 cl (8 fl oz)	40
63% Carbohydrate	6 g
7% Protein	1 g
30% Fat	1 g
CALCIUM	9 mg
IRON	Trace
SODIUM	9 mg

Place the chicken bones in a stockpot with 1.5 litres (2½ pints) of water and bring to the boil over medium-high heat. When the water comes to the boil, skim off the foam with a slotted spoon. Continue boiling and skimming for 5 minutes, or until most of the scum has risen and been removed. Add the carrots, onion, celery, garlic, bay leaf and peppercorns. Cover the pot, reduce the heat to medium low and simmer the stock for 2 hours. Remove the pot from the heat, uncover it and let the stock cool for about 30 minutes.

Strain the stock through a colander set over a large bowl; discard the solids. Cover and refrigerate the stock. When it is thoroughly chilled, remove any fat that has risen to the surface. Transfer the stock to storage jars or containers and refrigerate or freeze it. The stock will keep for a week in the refrigerator, but it should be brought to the boil and boiled for 5 minutes after 2 to 3 days, then cooled and returned to the refrigerator. The stock may be frozen for up to 1 month.   Makes about 1.5 litres (2½ pints)

QUICK CHICKEN-NOODLE SOUP

A steaming bowl of chicken soup is more than just an old wives' remedy
for treating colds or flu. The hot liquid can alleviate a sore throat, and
the vapour helps clear up head and chest congestion.

CALORIES per serving	195
73% Carbohydrate	36 g
14% Protein	7 g
13% Fat	3 g
CALCIUM	40 mg
IRON	2 mg
SODIUM	25 mg

1 litre (1¾ pints) low-sodium
   chicken stock (see page 134)
125 g (4 oz) carrots, julienned
125 g (4 oz) fine egg noodles

150 g (5 oz) fresh or frozen peas
2 tablespoons chopped parsley
½ teaspoon pepper

Bring the stock to the boil in a medium-sized saucepan over medium-high
heat. Add the carrots and cook for 2 to 3 minutes. Add the noodles, reduce
the heat to medium and cook for 3 minutes. Add the peas, parsley and pepper. Bring the soup to the boil, cook for 1 minute more and serve.

Makes 4 servings

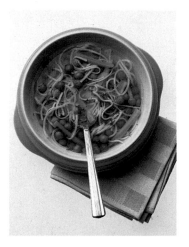

SWEET PEA SOUP

The peas in this meatless, low-sodium soup are a good source of
molybdenum, a trace mineral that helps the body metabolize nutrients.

2 teaspoons butter or margarine
125 g (4 oz) shallots, thinly sliced
1 teaspoon sugar
300 g (10 oz) fresh peas

12.5 cl (4 fl oz) low-sodium
   chicken stock, or vegetable stock
   (see page 134)

CALORIES per serving	110
63% Carbohydrate	18 g
18% Protein	5 g
19% Fat	2 g
CALCIUM	32 mg
IRON	2 mg
SODIUM	28 mg

Melt the butter in a medium-sized saucepan over medium heat. Add the shallots and sauté for 30 seconds. Add the sugar and cook, stirring, for 1 to 2
minutes, or until the sugar begins to caramelize. Add the peas, stock and 50
cl (16 fl oz) of water. Cover the pan, reduce the heat to low and simmer for 25
minutes. Remove the pan from the heat and let the soup cool for 20 minutes,
then purée the soup in a food processor or blender. Return the soup to the
pan, reheat it briefly over medium heat and serve.   Makes 4 servings

KALE AND MUSHROOM SOUP

Kale, like other dark green leafy vegetables, is a good non-dairy source of
calcium, which is essential primarily for the growth and maintenance of
bones and teeth.

2 garlic cloves, thinly sliced
2 teaspoons butter or margarine
350 g (12 oz) fresh kale, washed
   and cut into 5 mm (¼ inch)
   strips

175 g (6 oz) mushrooms, sliced
1 litre (1 ¾ pints) vegetable stock
   (see page 134)
¼ teaspoon pepper
Pinch of salt

CALORIES per serving	95
61% Carbohydrate	16 g
16% Protein	4 g
23% Fat	3 g
CALCIUM	148 mg
IRON	3 mg
SODIUM	259 mg

Sauté the garlic in the butter in a large saucepan over low heat for 2 to 3
minutes. Add the kale, mushrooms, stock, pepper and salt and bring to the
boil. Cover the pan, reduce the heat to low and simmer the mixture for 10 to
15 minutes, or until the vegetables are tender.   Makes 4 servings

PEAR AND CHICORY SALAD

In this fruit and vegetable salad, minimal amounts of quark and Gorgonzola take the place of bottled blue-cheese dressing, which has about 100 calories — and 10 grams of fat — per tablespoon.

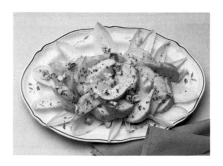

1 very ripe small pear (about 90 g/ 3 oz), plus 4 large William's pears (about 175 g/6 oz each)
3 tablespoons lemon juice
3 tablespoons apple juice
1 teaspoon sugar

1 tablespoon chopped parsley
1 tablespoon quark
175 g (6 oz) chicory, separated into leaves
30 g (1 oz) Gorgonzola cheese

CALORIES per serving	155
75% Carbohydrate	32 g
7% Protein	3 g
18% Fat	3 g
CALCIUM	68 mg
IRON	1 mg
SODIUM	107 mg

For the dressing, peel and core the small pear. Cut it into large chunks, place them in a small bowl and mash with a fork until smooth. Stir in 2 tablespoons of the lemon juice, the apple juice, sugar, parsley and quark; set aside. Halve, stem and core but do not peel the remaining pears. Cut them lengthwise into 5 mm (¼ inch) thick slices, place them in a medium-sized bowl and toss with the remaining lemon juice. Line a serving platter with the chicory leaves and arrange the pear slices on top. Crumble the cheese over the pears and dribble the dressing over the salad.   Makes 4 servings

TOMATO-RICE SOUP WITH BASIL

The brown rice in this dish has significantly more potassium, magnesium and fibre than does white rice, which is more processed.

1 kg (2 lb) fresh ripe tomatoes, or canned tomatoes, drained
250 g (8 oz) cooked brown rice (90 g/3 oz raw)
125 g (4 oz) celery, chopped
90 g (3 oz) onion, chopped
2 garlic cloves, chopped

4 tablespoons chopped fresh basil
3 tablespoons tomato paste
1 tablespoon sugar
Pinch of salt
¼ teaspoon pepper
1 bay leaf

CALORIES per serving	85
86% Carbohydrate	19 g
9% Protein	2 g
5% Fat	0.4 g
CALCIUM	39 mg
IRON	1 mg
SODIUM	105 mg

If using fresh tomatoes, core and quarter them. Place the tomatoes in a large non-reactive pan and add one third of the rice, the celery, onion, garlic, basil, tomato paste, sugar, salt, pepper, bay leaf and 1 litre (1¾ pints) of water. Bring to the boil over medium heat, then cover the pan, reduce the heat to low and simmer the soup for about 30 minutes, stirring occasionally and breaking up the tomatoes with the edge of the spoon.

Remove the pan from the heat, uncover it and allow the soup to cool for about 30 minutes; remove the bay leaf. Transfer the soup to a food processor or blender, in two batches if necessary, and process until puréed. Return the soup to the pan and stir in the remaining rice. Reheat the soup over medium heat, divide it among six bowls and serve.   Makes 6 servings

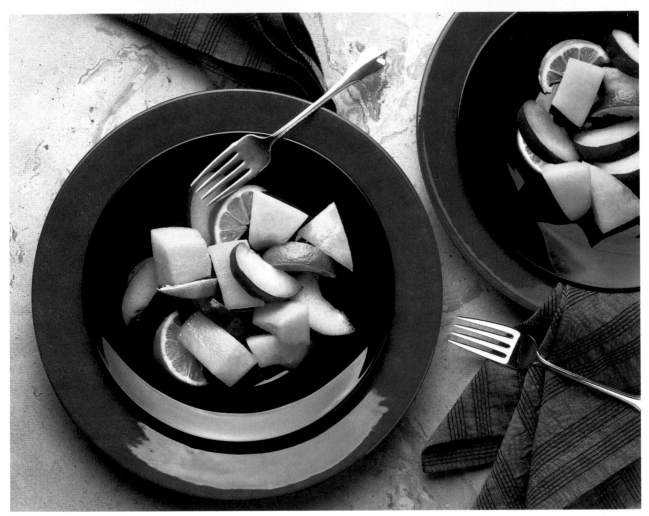

Plum-Cantaloupe Salad

Desserts

PLUM-CANTALOUPE SALAD

*Eating a fruit salad for dessert is a good way to increase your fluid intake
without stinting on the fibre, and the tartness of lime makes this salad
especially refreshing. The fruits supply a good amount of vitamins A and C
as well.*

CALORIES per serving	**75**
86% Carbohydrate	**18 g**
7% Protein	**1 g**
7% Fat	**0.5 g**
CALCIUM	**19 mg**
IRON	**Trace**
SODIUM	**11 mg**

One 1 kg (2 lb) cantaloupe melon   **½ lime**
250 g (8 oz) plums   **1 teaspoon pure maple syrup**

Halve and seed the melon; cut each half into three wedges. Remove the rind
and cut the flesh into 2.5 cm (1 inch) chunks. Halve and stone the plums; cut
the halves into 5 mm (¼ inch) thick wedges. Cut the lime half into 5 mm
(¼ inch) thick wedges. Place the fruit and maple syrup in a large bowl and
toss to combine, then cover and refrigerate overnight to allow the flavours to
blend. Serve chilled or at room temperature.   Makes 4 servings

CHOCOLATE BANANA CREAM

Made without eggs or cream, this mousse-like dessert is low in fat, making it a healthy substitute for ice cream or another pudding.

15 g (½ oz) plain chocolate
2 tablespoons sugar

2 bananas, peeled
35 cl (12 fl oz) plain low-fat yogurt

CALORIES per serving	150
71% Carbohydrate	28 g
13% Protein	5 g
16% Fat	3 g
CALCIUM	160 mg
IRON	Trace
SODIUM	60 mg

Heat the chocolate, sugar and 1 tablespoon of water in a small saucepan over very low heat, stirring constantly, until the chocolate is melted; remove the pan from the heat and set aside. Purée the bananas in a food processor or blender, add the yogurt and the chocolate mixture, and process for 5 to 10 seconds, scraping down the sides of the container with a rubber spatula. Divide the mixture among four dessert bowls and refrigerate for 2 to 3 hours, or until well chilled.   Makes 4 servings

WATERMELON-BLUEBERRY ICE

Watermelon, as its name suggests, is mostly water, actually 93 per cent by volume; blueberries average 83 per cent water.

1 kg (2 lb) watermelon
** (weighed with rind)**

450 g (15 oz) fresh blueberries
1 tablespoon lime juice

CALORIES per serving	115
87% Carbohydrate	27 g
5% Protein	2 g
8% Fat	1 g
CALCIUM	20 mg
IRON	1 mg
SODIUM	10 mg

Scoop the flesh of the watermelon into a large bowl; remove and discard the seeds. Place the watermelon flesh in a food processor or blender and process until liquefied; you should have about 55 cl (18 fl oz) of juice. Pour the juice into a shallow 20 cm (8 inch) pan. Process the blueberries until puréed, then stir the purée and the lime juice into the watermelon juice. Freeze the mixture for 2 to 3 hours, or until partially frozen.

Scrape the partially frozen ice into a bowl and break it up with a whisk, then return it to the pan and freeze it for another 3 to 4 hours, or until frozen solid. Let the ice thaw at room temperature for 15 to 30 minutes, or until slightly softened, before serving.   Makes 4 servings

PINEAPPLE CREAM

Fresh pineapple is an excellent source of vitamin C.

One 1 kg (2 lb) pineapple
12.5 cl (4 fl oz) plain low-fat
** yogurt**

1 teaspoon honey
1 teaspoon pure vanilla extract

CALORIES per serving	110
84% Carbohydrate	25 g
7% Protein	2 g
9% Fat	1 g
CALCIUM	64 mg
IRON	1 mg
SODIUM	22 mg

Using a large, heavy knife, cut the leaves from the pineapple, then quarter the fruit lengthwise. Run the knife along the inside of the rind to remove the flesh. For the cream, coarsely chop 75 g (2 ½ oz) of the pineapple flesh and purée it in a blender with the yogurt, honey and vanilla; set aside. Cut the remaining pineapple crosswise into 5 mm (¼ inch) thick triangles and place them in a large bowl. Add the pineapple cream and toss to combine. Cover the bowl and refrigerate for at least 4 hours, stirring occasionally, to allow the flavours to blend. Serve chilled or at room temperature.   Makes 4 servings

PINEAPPLE-ORANGE BARS

These virtually fat-free frozen bars are made without added sugar; the natural sweetness of the pineapple easily satisfies a sweet tooth.

One 300 g (10 oz) can crushed pineapple, in natural juice

Juice of 2 oranges (about 15 cl/ ¼ pint)

Stir the pineapple and its juice together with the orange juice in a medium-sized bowl. Divide the mixture among five ice lolly moulds or small paper cups. Freeze the bars for about 1 hour, or until partially frozen, then insert a lolly stick in the centre of each and freeze overnight, or until frozen solid. To unmould the bars, dip the moulds into hot water for about 5 seconds; if using paper cups, tear the edge of the cup and peel it off.   Makes 5 servings

CALORIES per serving	50
95% Carbohydrate	12 g
3% Protein	1 g
2% Fat	0.1 g
CALCIUM	12 mg
IRON	2 mg
SODIUM	1 mg

STRAWBERRY BUTTERMILK MOUSSE

Slightly less sour than yogurt and far healthier than cream, buttermilk makes a good basis for desserts.

3 tablespoons lemon juice

7 g (¼ oz) unflavoured gelatine

300 g (10 oz) strawberries

2 bananas, peeled

25 cl (8 fl oz) buttermilk

1 tablespoon honey

Heat the lemon juice in a small saucepan over low heat for 2 minutes. Sprinkle in the gelatine and stir until it is completely dissolved; remove the pan from the heat and set aside. Wash and hull the strawberries. Purée the bananas and half of the strawberries in a food processor or blender. Add the gelatine mixture, buttermilk and honey, and process for 5 to 10 seconds, scraping down the sides of the container with a rubber spatula. Coarsely chop the remaining strawberries and add them to the mixture, then spoon it into a 1 litre (2 pint) soufflé dish or six individual dessert dishes. Cover loosely and refrigerate overnight.   Makes 6 servings

CALORIES per serving	90
79% Carbohydrate	21 g
14% Protein	4 g
7% Fat	1 g
CALCIUM	66 mg
IRON	Trace
SODIUM	22 mg

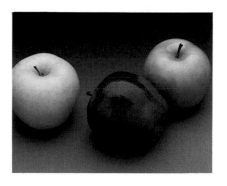

THREE-APPLE MÉLANGE

Unpeeled apples are high in pectin, a type of dietary fibre that can help lower blood cholesterol.

2 each Granny Smith, Red Delicious and Golden Delicious apples (about 850 g/1¾ lb total weight)

1 tablespoon lemon juice

25 cl (8 fl oz) buttermilk

125 g (4 oz) sultanas

2 tablespoons brown sugar

½ teaspoon grated lemon rind

Pinch of ground cinnamon

Core but do not peel the apples and cut them into 4 cm (1½ inch) chunks. Place the apples in a medium-sized bowl, add the lemon juice and toss to coat the apples; set aside. For the sauce, combine the buttermilk, sultanas, sugar and lemon rind in a small bowl, stirring until the sugar is completely dissolved. Divide the apples among six plates, pour some of the sauce over each serving and dust with the cinnamon.   Makes 6 servings

CALORIES per serving	155
90% Carbohydrate	38 g
5% Protein	2 g
5% Fat	1 g
CALCIUM	69 mg
IRON	1 mg
SODIUM	47 mg

Beverages

WATERMELON-GRAPE SLUSH

When you make your own cooling fruit slush, you avoid the excessive sugar found in commercial ice slush drinks which are made with sugar-based syrups.

750 g (1½ lb) seedless red grapes, washed and stemmed	**12 fresh mint leaves, plus 4 sprigs for garnish**
1 kg (2 lb) watermelon	**Crushed ice (see note)**

Place the grapes in a food processor or blender and process until puréed. Pour the purée into a large strainer placed over a bowl and press the pulp with a rubber spatula to extract as much juice as possible; you should have about 50 cl (16 fl oz) of juice. Discard the pulp. Scoop the flesh of the watermelon into a bowl and remove and discard the seeds. Place the watermelon flesh in a food processor or blender and process until liquefied; you should have about 50 cl (16 fl oz) of juice. Add the watermelon juice and mint leaves to the grape juice, cover the bowl and refrigerate the mixture for 2 to 3 hours to allow the flavours to blend. Remove and discard the mint. To serve, scoop a teacup of crushed ice into each of four dessert glasses and pour 25 cl (8 fl oz) of the watermelon-grape juice into each glass. Garnish with the mint sprigs.　　　　　　　　　Makes 4 servings

Note: to crush ice, place ice cubes in double-thickness heavy-duty polythene bags (such as dustbin bags) and pound with a mallet or meat pounder until the ice is broken into almond-sized pieces, then place it in a food processor or blender and process for 15 to 30 seconds, or until finely crushed.

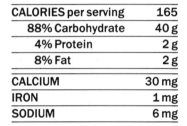

CALORIES per serving	165
88% Carbohydrate	40 g
4% Protein	2 g
8% Fat	2 g
CALCIUM	30 mg
IRON	1 mg
SODIUM	6 mg

Watermelon-Grape Slush

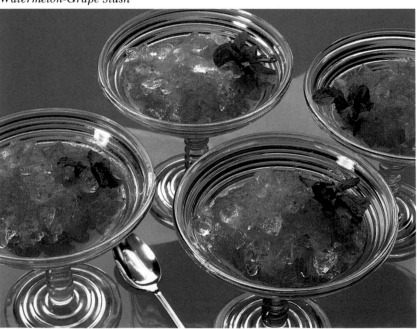

CITRUSADE

Quench your thirst with this refreshing drink and you will get almost 200 milligrams of vitamin C — nearly seven times the daily requirement.

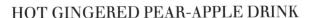

2 large pink grapefruits (about 1.5 kg/3 lb)
4 juicy oranges (about 1.1 kg/ 2¼ lb)

1 lemon
1 lime
1 tablespoon finely chopped fresh basil

Halve and squeeze the grapefruits, oranges, lemon and lime. Strain the juices into a medium-sized bowl; discard the pulp and seeds. Stir the basil into the juice. Serve the citrusade over ice in tall glasses.   Makes 2 servings

Note: to get the maximum amount of juice, warm the citrus fruits slightly, then roll them on a work surface, pressing with your palm, before cutting them.

CALORIES per serving	185
92% Carbohydrate	45 g
5% Protein	3 g
3% Fat	1 g
CALCIUM	56 mg
IRON	1 mg
SODIUM	5 mg

HOT GINGERED PEAR-APPLE DRINK

A thermos flask of this drink, preferably made with fresh apple juice, is a perfect warmer for autumn sports outings.

4 William's pears (about 750 g/ 1½ lb)
1 litre (1¾ pints) unsweetened apple juice

30 g (1 oz) fresh ginger root, sliced, plus additional ginger slices for garnish (optional)

Peel, core and stem the pears and cut them into 2.5 cm (1 inch) chunks. Place the pears, apple juice and ginger in a medium-sized non-reactive saucepan and bring to the boil over medium heat. Cover the pan, reduce the heat to low and simmer for 5 to 10 minutes, or until the pears are tender. Remove the ginger. Let the mixture cool slightly, then purée it in a food processor or blender. Reheat the drink over low heat and garnish with fresh ginger slices if desired. The drink can be refrigerated and reheated later; it will keep for 2 days in a covered jar in the refrigerator.   Makes 4 servings

CALORIES per serving	210
95% Carbohydrate	53 g
1% Protein	1 g
4% Fat	1 g
CALCIUM	35 mg
IRON	1 mg
SODIUM	8 mg

SPICED APPLE-GRAPEFRUIT TEA

Caffeine, found in coffee, tea and some soft drinks, may be a contributory factor in osteoporosis, but this tea is caffeine-free.

1 apple-spice herbal tea bag
1 large pink grapefruit (about 750 g/1 ½ lb)

1 teaspoon honey

Place the tea bag in a teapot, add 25 cl (8 fl oz) of boiling water and set aside to steep for about 10 minutes. Meanwhile, halve the grapefruit and squeeze enough juice to measure 25 cl (8 fl oz). Strain the juice into a saucepan, add the honey and bring the mixture to a simmer over low heat. Discard the tea bag, add the grapefruit juice to the tea and stir to blend. Pour the tea into two mugs and serve.   Makes 2 servings

CALORIES per serving	60
94% Carbohydrate	15 g
4% Protein	1 g
2% Fat	0.1 g
CALCIUM	15 mg
IRON	Trace
SODIUM	1 mg

ACKNOWLEDGEMENTS

The editors wish to thank Irena Hoare and Norma MacMillan.
Index prepared by Ian Tucker.

PHOTOGRAPHY CREDIT

All photographs by Steven Mays, Rebus, Inc.

ILLUSTRATION CREDITS

Page 8, illustration: Tammi Colichio, Brian Sisco; page 11, illustration: David Flaherty; page 12, illustration: David Flaherty; page 14, chart: Brian Sisco; page 16, illustration: David Flaherty; page 17, illustration: David Flaherty; page 21, illustration: Tammi Colichio; page 25, illustration: Tammi Colichio; page 28, illustration: David Flaherty, chart: Brian Sisco; page 31, illustration: Tammi Colichio, chart: Brian Sisco; page 37, illustration: Dana Burns-Pizer; pages 40-43, illustrations: Dana Burns-Pizer; page 63, illustration: Dana Burns-Pizer; pages 66-67, illustrations: Dana Burns-Pizer; page 95, illustration: Dana Burns-Pizer.

Typeset by A.J. Latham Limited, Dunstable,
Bedfordshire, England
Printed by GEA, Milan and bound by GEP,
Cremona, Italy

INDEX